CHARLES MOSELEY

Why We Shouldnt Drink Alcohol

This book sets out in clear terms how alcohol is detrimental to our health and wellbeing

Contact:

charles@i-modify.org

+447587428687

www.whyweshouldntdrinkalcohol.co.uk

First edition

ISBN: 9798730587854

This book was professionally typeset on Reedsy.
Find out more at reedsy.com

Contents

1

Introduction

It is important that I say up front that I am not a doctor or a scientist, or an expert in the field of addiction. I am not qualified to explain differences in brain chemistry, or the precise levels of alcohol that cause certain effects in various parts of the body. I have never worked with patients in a medical setting, seeing exactly what harm they have caused themselves by drinking heavily. I'm not familiar with the typical diseases that afflict drinkers or how to diagnose them. I would never try to offer medical advice or treatment or pretend to know about anything that would ordinarily fall to a doctor. Doctors understand illnesses, diseases and injuries, and they know how to treat them. Doctors are qualified to give out medical advice, and I am not.

Scientists understand the detailed way that alcohol works on the body. They come up with various theories based on what they see in the lab, in the patients that they work with, and they review existing studies and evidence from research and trials. I am not a scientist. Scientists look at the workings of the brain, geneticists consider the effect of different genetic profiles, and various other disciplines use their collective understanding of biological factors to understand how alcohol affects us. Scientists, doctors, psychiatrists and addiction specialists have collectively contributed to the guidance that keeps us all safe from the potential harms of drinking. I am not one of them.

I drank alcohol regularly from age 14 until a few years ago when I happened across a couple of interesting texts that made me think differently about alcohol. One day I was a drinker that believed what we all believe about alcohol, the next I was a non-drinker, with a different set of beliefs (If you are not keen on reading a whole book and you prefer to jump straight to these beliefs go to the short chapter called Beliefs to see them). Now I don't miss drinking and I don't feel deprived if I can't drink.

When I take an honest look back at my 35 years of drinking alcohol I don't see any of it as positive. I had some great nights out but generally the promise of the night was great, and in any evening I only behaved well up to the second drink. The list of my transgressions is long and I am embarrassed at my behaviour on so many occasions, from rude comments to aggression, selfishness, arguments and generally acting less well than if I was sober. Like most people that drink too much I was mostly boring and annoying, but at the same time I believed I was hilarious and charming. On the mornings when I was hungover I also had a sense that I had lost control the night before. I experienced a nagging feeling that my plan for the evening had been derailed by alcohol. Even though I believed I had to drink at social events, time and time again I spent the next morning reviewing the evening wondering what caused me to behave badly, and to drink too much. I often drank enough to negatively impact my personality. Like every human I am a naturally social person, a great communicator and a happy positive person. I wasn't those things when I was drinking. I would have been a better version of me without the alcohol.

Once I had spent some time understanding how alcohol really affected me, I found that my beliefs about drinking changed very quickly. My alcohol intake quickly went from substantial to nothing with no difficulty. I didn't need to turn to complicated scientific theories or medical advice to figure out what was wrong with me, it was obviously the alcohol that was a problem. Now that I have a different set of beliefs about alcohol I realise that the things I know now are the same things I knew before I started drinking. When I was a child I could enjoy social events without alcohol, enjoyed dinner without wine, and went to parties for the social interaction and the fun of interacting with other kids. Why did I start drinking as a teenager? Because other drinkers recruited me and told me I couldn't socialise without a drink in my hand. I'm embarrassed to say that it took me 35 years to realise that I was fine without a drink, and to realise that I was a better person in my natural state.

I am not a scientist or a doctor or a psychologist or an addiction specialist but I don't drink alcohol, and the majority of individuals that practice in these fields do. Instead of pretending I am qualified to give out medical or scientific advice this book is my attempt to explain in common sense why we shouldn't drink. Drinking alcohol goes against our natural instincts for health and wellbeing. It negatively impacts our social interaction and it upsets our body's in-built controls and safety systems.

Whatever your current level of alcohol consumption, I hope you find this book thought provoking. It is not designed as a self help book, more of a review of the factors that cause people to drink, and the mistaken beliefs that all drinkers hold about alcohol.

2

Our natural selves

Picture a herd of antelope in their multitudes and you should be visualising lots of brown, furry animals with horns. Antelope are all the same size and shape and they have evolved to suit the natural environment they live in. Which of these antelopes is depressed? Which of these antelopes is stressed? Which one is massively fat because he gorges on cake and chocolate? Which of these antelopes is drinking too much whiskey or smoking cigarettes? Which of these antelopes has breast cancer? Which of these antelopes needs to take steroids because the pollutants in the air cause her lungs not to work? Obviously none of them, all antelopes are happy being antelopes in their natural environment. They don't get fat or die of cancer because they eat the right food, they stick together and exist as a herd and they don't use addictive drugs because they're antelope. Every so often a slow old antelope may not be able to get enough food or may get eaten by predators but essentially antelopes are happy and healthy doing antelope stuff.

In the same way that antelope are happy doing what is natural to antelope, humans are happy and healthy doing human stuff. We have evolved to suit our environment and like antelope, if we focus on what is good for us and we don't damage or pollute our surroundings we should be healthy and happy. Unfortunately in our desire for progress and in the name of profit we have put a lot of effort into creating food and drinks that we don't need and that have the potential for harm, medication and remedies that we tell each other are necessary for our wellbeing, and inventions that appear to provide a benefit while harming us and our environment.

Like the members of every species, each individual human is essentially the same as every other human. We are all 100% perfect and amazing. Evolution has made us what we are and provided us with the most sophisticated systems and controls to keep us safe and well. We have evolved to suit our environment and we thrive in almost all corners of the world. Our natural self is phenomenal and like every other human each of us can communicate, collaborate and socialise to achieve tasks and to live successfully in groups. Sometimes though, we forget how perfect we are and believe some of the marketing and falsehoods that our fellow humans tell us, to make us believe we are deficient in some way.

We have a highly sophisticated reflex system that keeps us safe when we fall over, or we feel pain or we get close to extreme heat, or sense danger. Our central nervous system and peripheral nervous system work together to relay messages to and from the brain and body. Our systems and controls tell us everything is OK. Like the dashboard in the cockpit of a plane we have a constant set of indicators that we can ignore when everything is fine, but that warn us if something is wrong and we need to take action. Are we experiencing any pain, do we need to jerk a hand away from something dangerous, is there something causing us irritation, has something stung us or bitten us, is there something wrong with us? Are we too hot, or too cold, are we short of food or water? And think of the incredible ability of our body to regulate our own body temperature using sweat to cool us. Every human is currently the same temperature as every other human on the planet. And when we are too hot we know that something is wrong. We may have a virus or an infection. These signals and controls are phenomenal.

Every human on the planet also has an amazing ability to communicate with any other human. Because we are all members of the same species we have a common facial language that is universally understood. A smile is a smile in every culture, a frown means the same to everybody on the planet and all seven billion of us raise our eyebrows in surprise when something surprises us. Each of us is amazing and the proof is in our success as a species. We have taken over the world and we're doing brilliantly. All we have to do to be happy is to do what is natural to us. Eat the right food, do enough exercise, sleep well, live with purpose, avoid stress and be social. The inhabitants of Okinawa, Japan exemplify this philosophy, and as a result they live longer than any other people on earth. They embody natural living, and a simple philosophy that results in a long life. They have a strong social network, eat fruit and vegetables, exercise regularly, enjoy the outdoors and sleep well[1]. This simple recipe for success, which works to keep us alive for a long time, seems to be forgotten by so many of us.

The things that cause us harm are unnatural and external such as pollutants in the environment or substances that we were not designed to consume and that are poisonous to us. Eating junk food, or processed food, eating too much sugar or fat, eating too much meat, inhaling poisonous smoke, taking drugs, and drinking alcohol are typical of the things that shorten our lives and cause us to be less healthy. To live long healthy lives we need to understand what is natural and appropriate for us, and reject the things that are offered to us and that go against nature. Nature has made us happy in our natural state. Each of us can improve our mood by giving up the practices that go against nature, and we should become happier by adopting more natural activities.

Nature provides solutions to a lot of what we need and allows us to challenge some of the pseudo-science that is used to sell us products we don't need, or that are not good for us. Science is amazing when it really solves mankind's problems, for example by producing vaccines, propelling us into space, solving our energy needs and improving our daily lives. But science is

---

[1] Dan Buettner, *Okinawa Japan, Secrets of the world's longest-living women*, Blue Zones. https://www.bluezones.com/exploration/okinawa-japan/ [17.3.21]

often used to generate profit by giving us advice that in some cases goes against nature. Science is used to sell us lotions and potions as part of highly sophisticated marketing that plays into our worries about our diet, about getting older or about the way we care for our bodies. Pharmaceutical companies use science and medical language to tell us that their products will make us look younger or more beautiful, or improve our skin or our hair, presenting us as deficient in our natural state. Their messaging is that without their products our natural self has shortcomings. Because we are perfect in our natural state and provided we are healthy and have our basic needs fulfilled then we don't need to subscribe to these offerings. The aim generally is to sell us something we don't need.

The promotion of suntan lotion is a good example. For around six million years our species, and other related species, have been hairless[2], and in that time nature and evolution has caused us to develop an incredible system for dealing with the sun. Sunlight is a form of radiation that causes our skin to change colour based on how long we have been in the sun for and how regularly we are in the sun. It is painful to be sunburnt and the more burnt we get, the more pain we experience. As kids, our mothers allow us in the sun but not for too long. As adults, the colour/pain system allows us to be in the sun for just the right amount of time using the natural system that is inherent in all of us. It warns us of the danger of too much radiation. We know what people who have been out for too long look like - bright red in colour, blisters and angry skin that gives off heat.

The first suntan protection was developed to protect military personnel stationed in the Pacific during the second world war, where they couldn't easily stay out of the sun. Science provided a solution to a specific problem and stepped in to help. In daily life humans had until then covered up, or

---

[2] Shizuyo Sutou, *Hairless mutation: a driving force of humanization from a human–ape common ancestor by enforcing upright walking while holding a baby with both hands*, National Library of Medicine. https://pubmed.ncbi.nlm.nih.gov/22404045/ [17.3.21]

7

gone indoors to avoid burning in the sun. The scientific solution that was developed for military use became Coppertone in the early 50s and the suntan industry was born.[3] We now spend $8.5 billion globally on suntan lotion each year[4]. When Piz Buin, the manufacturer of expensive suntan lotion says, "Whether you call it sunscreen, sun cream or sun protection, one thing is for sure – it's not optional."[5] we should be able to question that. Suntan lotion isn't necessary, and our natural system works well to protect us. Nature has given us a sophisticated system for regulating our exposure to sunlight. Holidaymakers that use suntan lotion end up lying in the sun for hours, a behaviour that goes against nature. Sophisticated marketing that uses words like "protection" has embedded the idea that we can't do without these products. Consumers can allow themselves to be taken in by the science peddled by the suntan lotion industry or they can choose the natural option and stay safe by covering up.

Alcohol has a lot in common with the lotions and potions that are sold to us unnecessarily. Drinkers hold a set of beliefs about the alcohol they consume that keeps them drinking, and the experts that we rely on for guidance about our intake of alcohol advise us to consume it, albeit in moderate amounts. Drinking alcohol has been normalised by the people that consume it and it is such a part of our lives that it seems natural. Drinkers believe that they are deficient without a drink in their hand, that they can't function socially, or celebrate without booze. The belief is supported by the scientists and experts that provide guidance to us and whose ideas about alcohol have filtered down into our collective consciousness. Their guidance is biased, advising us that drinking in moderation is normal, because the authors of the studies are drinkers. Nature tells us that we shouldn't drink it by warning us using our control systems. Scientists say we should drink it. We all have the good sense

---

[3] Sunscreen, Wikipedia, https://en.wikipedia.org/wiki/Sunscreen [17.3.21]

[4] M Ridder, Global market size of sunscreen cream 2019-2024, Statista, https://www.statista.com/statistics/866356/ [17.3.21]

[5] Piz Buin marketing text https://www.boots.com/piz-buin [17.3.21]

to know when something that we have been told we need goes against nature.

3

Nature versus alcohol

I have a fantastic picture of my son at 10 years old. He's in school uniform, leaning on a wall and he has a cheeky grin on his face. I took the picture when he was on his way home from school with me. He looks like a healthy, happy, child. Just thinking of the picture makes me smile. You can probably picture a similar child if you have children of your own, or know of a relative or maybe a cousin or sibling. If you have a picture of a child in mind, you are picturing a healthy, happy and natural human before they get to adulthood. Now imagine the same picture of the child with a half empty bottle of whiskey in his or her hand and think about the way it makes you feel. Most of us would be disgusted at the image. A child shouldn't be drinking whiskey, and we should be appalled at the idea of it happening. Children exemplify what it is to be a natural human - we like them free of unnatural substances. The idea of children drinking it is abhorrent to us because we know that whiskey is extremely bad for children. If offered to them, they would smell it and push it away, taste it and look horrified that someone was encouraging them to drink it, and if they swallowed a small amount their balance and coordination would be affected. A bit more would cause them to vomit up the foul substance and if you forced them to drink too much they would collapse and die. Whiskey is poisonous to children. All alcohol is poisonous to children. And if it's poisonous to children it is poisonous to adults. Every rational, caring person would be appalled at the idea of giving alcohol to a child, and if we apply high standards in the way we treat our children shouldn't we also apply the same standards to ourselves as adults?

Over millions of years all animals' and humans' taste systems have evolved to make sure that we eat things that are good for us and keep us safe. When we smell or taste fresh fruit we experience a pleasant sensation because it is exactly what we should be eating. When we smell or taste rotten fruit it tastes off, bad, poisonous. We sense that something is wrong with it and we turn our noses up and the disgust registers on our face. The delicious taste of fresh green grapes is perfect but if the same fruit is decaying it doesn't appeal. Nature has given us an amazing set of controls and mechanisms to keep us safe. Our sense of taste, smell and our eyesight and experience of eating the right things means that when we encounter the wrong things we are repelled.

Alcoholic drinks taste nasty because they are the result of fruit, or grain, rotting. A percentage of the drink is made up of highly toxic ethanol, and the remainder is fruit or grain juice that has gone off. Alcohol is poisonous to humans and we are not meant to drink it. The unpleasant taste indicates that this is not meant for us. Alcohol has an acrid smell in its pure form and when we smell it we recognise it as the smell of hospitals and medical facilities. This is because it kills germs, and is used as a powerful disinfectant, floor cleaner and a hand sanitiser. The reason that alcohol lasts for years in a sealed bottle is that it is a poisonous chemical that kills germs.

Our social drinking tends to be based around drinks that comprise between five and 15% alcohol. We mix the foul tasting ethanol with sickly sweet fruit juice or sugary soft drinks to mask the taste. Think of a vodka and coke or whiskey and ginger ale as typical examples – the neat spirit tastes foul on its own but diluted into the sweet sickly drink the spirit becomes palatable. I could mask the taste of my own piss if I diluted it in Coca Cola at 10% but I really wouldn't want to. When we drink shots of strong alcohol drinkers grimace at the taste. The grimace is because the taste is disgusting. The alcohol tastes disgusting because it is toxic. Drinkers are drinking a poison that the body does not want us to drink. The word intoxicated isn't a positive - the consumption of a toxic substance is bad.

There are wine producers and sellers that will tell us that one vineyard produces wine that tastes better than another vineyard, or that wine produced in 1963 tastes better than wine produced in 1983. Wine experts will waffle on about the qualities of a certain bouquet, and advise us to drink certain wines with certain foods. Drinkers may believe that older wines taste better if they have been stored for years. They may believe that fizzy rotten grape juice is worth buying for £50 a bottle, or that old wine is worth thousands per bottle. For pseudo wine buffs that believe all this nonsense here's an easy test to see if the wine that they believe tastes nice really does taste nice. Pour a glass for a young child and ask them to review it - they will, truthfully, tell you it is foul. Maybe pour a saucer-full for a dog or cat and see if they lap up the acrid liquid. Kids and animals will reject wine because it tastes like grape juice that has rotted. Ah, but apparently to enjoy wine, we have to 'acquire the taste', which actually means that to become a drinker each new recruit has had to learn to put up with the foul taste of alcohol, and to convince the body to hold down the poison, working against the body's natural defences.

The same substance that is in our drinks is used by the chemical industry in a number of products. Here is an overview from MSDSOnline, a website that covers activity in the chemical sectors, and which describes ethanol as "Versatile, Common and Potentially Dangerous,":

> "Ethanol is a colorless, volatile and highly flammable liquid that has a slight odor. Ethanol has been around for centuries, having been discovered as a by-product of fermentation... Ethanol is part of the hydroxyl group, which makes it a substructure of the water molecule. Because of its incredible versatility, ethanol mixes very well with other solvents and water, as well as chlorides and hydrocarbons. Being this versatile, ethanol is used for a great many things – but it can also be quite dangerous...

Where is Ethanol used in the Home or Workplace?

Ethanol is most commonly used in alcoholic beverages; however, there are many more household and workplace items in which it is used:

- *Manufacture of varnishes*
- *Nail polish remover*
- *Perfumes*
- *Biofuel*
- *Gasoline additive*
- *Preservative for biochemical samples*
- *Medicines*
- *Household cleaning products*
- *Beauty products*
- *Various solvents*

Hazards Associated with Using Ethanol

Even though ethanol is very commonly used, it is a dangerous chemical. As previously mentioned, it is highly flammable; as such, it has exact flash points which are important to know when using it. While ethanol is consumed when drinking alcoholic beverages, consuming ethanol alone can cause coma and death. Ethanol may also be a carcinogenic; studies are still being done to determine this. However, ethanol is a toxic chemical and should be treated and handled as such, whether at work or in the home."[6]

To recap, the chemical that we drink, that makes up 13% of wine, 5% of beer and around 40% of whiskey causes coma and death, is carcinogenic and is described as a toxic chemical. It is used in household cleaning products, varnishes, it gets polish off nails (and nail polish is very difficult to get off!), and it is put into petrol because it burns. No wonder it tastes foul.

---

[6] *Ethanol: Versatile, Common and Potentially Dangerous,* MSDSonline.
 https://www.msdsonline.com/2014/04/21/ethanol-versatile-common-and-potentially-dangerous/ [17.3.21]

When we smell and taste alcohol we get a warning from our senses that we shouldn't drink it but of course our peers encourage us to put up with the taste and man up, or learn to drink it. Luckily for us nature has also given us some extra facilities for dealing with the threat of a poison. When we start our drinking, at some point we drink too much and our stomach rejects the poison. Our body vomits the contents of our stomach in an attempt to keep us safe. This isn't a conscious decision, it's a reflex action and an example of our natural safety mechanism trying to protect us. Do drinkers stop consuming alcohol at this point? No, because our peers tell us we have to learn to keep it down.

As if the taste and the smell and the vomiting weren't enough, when we first drink we feel alarmingly unsteady as the poisonous alcohol causes us to lose control of our balance and our physical control. The dizzying unsteady effect is the result of consuming a powerful anesthetic and again, it should put us off. We lose control of our speech, our judgement and our emotions but still we persevere as we learn to tolerate this poisonous substance. Our determination to drink an addictive poisonous chemical means we have to work hard to ignore nature's warning signs and even though our body and brain tell us this is a substance that is alien to us, we persevere to ensure we learn how to drink the substance.

4

Water management

Humans have a very sophisticated system to manage our water intake and storage. In our daily lives work and play requires us to sweat to stay cool. Our natural system for water management includes a reserve that we hold, to ensure that when we work especially hard, for example when we run or play sport, we have enough water to keep us safe. The reserve is there so that we can continue to produce sweat for an extended period of time and the reserve of water is connected to the senses that signal to us that we should drink. If our reserve of water needs topping up we feel thirsty and we gulp down water to top up the tank. This natural in-built system is extremely sophisticated and is designed to keep us hydrated in all conditions. When we drink alcohol though we cause this system to malfunction. The alcohol interferes with our natural controls so that when we drink we cause our body to purge the reserve water that we hold. It is ejected to our bladder and we piss it out. Drinkers will know the experience of weeing a lot more than usual, and a lot more than they have just consumed, after a few drinks. A drinker after a few pints, or glasses of wine, now has a depleted water reserve, which has the potential to be dangerous. The obvious solution is to drink a lot of water before going to bed, which is common practice among drinkers. This does not work though, because the drinker goes to bed with enough alcohol in his or her system to still interfere with the water reserve. The water consumed at bedtime goes straight to the bladder. The next day the hungover drinker is bound to feel thirsty because the reserve tank is depleted, and the parched throat and dry mouth is the result. The next day following a drinking session, vigorous exercise has the potential to be dangerous because there is no reserve water available in the system.[7]

---

7   *Why does alcohol make you pee more?*, Drinkaware. https://www.drinkaware.co.uk/facts/health-effects-of-alcohol/effects-on-the-body/why-does-alcohol-make-you-pee-more [17.3.21]

5

Hangovers

The day after drinking, drinkers get another reminder of the poison we consumed last night. We wake up feeling tired, even though we slept for a long time, hungover and lethargic. We don't operate at our best when we are hungover and the combination of a headache, dehydration and feeling mentally and physically worse for wear tells us that the substance we consumed last night was very bad for us. Do we listen to our bodies at this point and stop drinking?

When we consume alcohol our amazing in-built protection system recognises the substance as a dangerous anesthetic and reacts by producing the stress hormone, cortisol. This is designed to keep us alert during times when we are in danger. Cortisol is one of our fight-or-flight hormones and is released when we are in a dangerous or threatening situation. The day after we consume alcohol drinkers will have an increased level of cortisol in their system and this makes them feel anxious and edgy. On top of the general lethargy, tiredness, headache and the dry mouth, that are the result of consuming a poisonous toxic chemical, drinkers feel heightened anxiety the day after drinking because of the increased levels of cortisol.

To recap, nature has given every human on the planet a set of reflexes and controls to keep us safe from harm. When we drink alcohol, our body reacts by giving us signals to let us know that we are causing ourselves potential harm. To become a drinker we have had to teach our poor, perfect, natural body to tolerate the poisonous substance, while ignoring the signals and forcing our reflexes to not react. We shouldn't allow alcohol to become a controlling aspect of our lives and yet in our early drinking we refuse to listen to nature, ignoring the warnings to learn to tolerate alcohol. As we continue to drink we still experience the hangovers, the anxiety and the detrimental effects of alcohol but instead of rejecting booze we buy into a set of false beliefs about alcohol, and the reasons for drinking it.

6

Pressure

It goes against nature to consume alcohol but there are a number of powerful forces that work to recruit new drinkers, to keep drinkers drinking, and to ensure that we maintain beliefs about the need to drink. The alcohol industry has an obvious interest in maintaining the status quo. It is extremely powerful and derives huge profits from selling a harmful over-priced product to us, presented as something that is supposed to show how sophisticated we are when we drink it. The alcohol industry though has the extra power of a huge volunteer force - the drinkers that consume its product. This massive population of drinkers backs up the alcohol industry's marketing by promoting booze and pressuring people into drinking. Does the media portray alcohol as a nasty addictive drug that causes harm to the people who drink it? Of course not, it represents it in a largely positive light and supports the alcohol industry. The powerful combination of marketing, media representation and billions of drinkers creates enormous pressure on drinkers.

Marketing pressure

EUCAM, The European Centre for Monitoring Alcohol Marketing, exists to monitor alcohol marketing and is independent from the alcohol industry. In 2014 it produced a report entitled *The seven key messages of the alcohol industry*, which highlights the way that the alcohol industry promotes drinking. It includes this no nonsense content:

> *The industry does not draw attention to the fact that alcohol (ethanol) is a detrimental, toxic, carcinogenic and addictive substance that is foreign to the body... Chemically, alcohol is a hard drug—a substance harmful to the body, which like heroin, can cause physical and mental dependence. The reality of the negative health effects is in direct contradiction to the industry's depiction of the consumer as responsible, social, happy and celebrating life with alcohol. Alcohol is carcinogenic... No safe limit of alcohol use has been identified in relation with cancer.*[8]

The Lancet's study, *Alcohol use and burden for 195 countries and territories, 1990–2016,* found that "Alcohol use is a leading risk factor for global disease burden and causes substantial health loss. We found that the risk of all-cause mortality, and of cancers specifically, rises with increasing levels of consumption, and the level of consumption that minimises health loss is zero. These results suggest that alcohol control policies might need to be revised worldwide, refocusing on efforts to lower overall population-level consumption."[9]

These two agencies that are not funded by the alcohol industry have concluded quite simply that "no safe limit of alcohol use has been identified," and "the level of consumption that minimises health loss is zero." This is straightforward and clear. Alcohol is dangerous, so don't drink it. But the alcohol industry, through a variety of methods including marketing, lobbying, press activities and sponsorship wants to continue to make big profits from

---

[8] *The Seven Key Messages of the Alcohol Industry, Information for everyone who wants to be aware of the real intentions of the alcohol industry,* EUCAM. http://eucam.info/wp-content/uploads/2014/04/seven_key_messages_of_the_alcohol_industry.pdf [17.3.21]

[9] M G Griswold et al. *Alcohol use and burden for 195 countries and territories, 1990–2016: a systematic analysis for the Global Burden of Disease Study 2016,* The Lancet https://www.thelancet.com/journals/lancet/article/PIIS0140-6736(18)31310-2/ [17.3.21]

selling alcohol. According to EUCAM "The alcohol industry... want to present the image of alcohol exclusively as a tasty and healthy product. From the perspective of the alcohol industry, consumption is a natural part of a modern healthy lifestyle and in order to portray this image they often neglect to inform the consumer of the disadvantages of alcohol consumption."[10] It points to one of the key messages repeated by the alcohol industry: "Alcohol is a tasty drink that is prepared with craftsmanship; the 'natural origin' of beer counts, wine is particularly beneficial for body and spirit, and with liquor, the age-long tradition guarantees the quality."

It is no surprise that the alcohol industry lies about its product. Like the tobacco industry, it sells a poisonous, harmful, addictive drug as a sophisticated product, apparently created by craftsmen and women, designed to convey heritage and tradition. Unlike tobacco the marketing of alcohol isn't nearly as tightly controlled, and the bottles don't have to convey warning labels. Imagine if a bottle of champagne had to carry a label saying "this wine is addictive. One glass will cause you to want to drink again." Picture a bottle of gin with a warning, "if you drink this entire bottle you could die." The marketing is to be expected, but the alcohol industry has another trick up its sleeve to ensure that its product continues to be drunk, and that is its funding of seemingly independent bodies that provide helpful advice to consumers about managing their intake.

Drinkaware describes itself as "an independent UK-wide alcohol education charity, funded largely by voluntary and unrestricted donations from UK alcohol producers, retailers and supermarkets. The Trust is governed independently and works in partnership with others to help reduce alcohol-related harm by helping people make better choices about their drinking."[11] It sounds noble to want to reduce alcohol-related harm but Drinkaware is funded by the drinks industry so clearly wants people to continue to

---

[10] *The Seven Key Messages of the Alcohol Industry*, EUCAM

[11] Drinkaware. https://www.drinkaware.co.uk/about-us [17.3.21]

drink. EUCAM and the authors of the study quoted in the Lancet have been very clear that alcohol is dangerous, and that the safe level is zero, but the massively powerful, global alcohol industry uses pseudo-independent groups to convince drinkers that they should drink moderate amounts. This has worked so well that it is nigh on impossible to find any reliable voices condemning alcohol, but it is also the view of almost all drinkers who continue to believe that a moderate amount of alcohol is beneficial.

The annual marketing spend globally by alcohol corporations is massive. David H.Jernigan of the PhD Center on Alcohol Marketing and Youth Department of Health, Behavior and Society, Johns Hopkins Bloomberg School of Public Health reported in his study of alcohol marketing that the traditional advertising spend in the US by just five alcohol corporations was $5.5 billion in 2010, and that alcohol companies feature in the top 10 spenders on advertising in many countries worldwide including Japan and Singapore.[12] In the UK we see advertising everywhere including sponsorship of sports at every level. Wine and beer is promoted to us constantly and alcohol companies support the film and TV industry, for example Heineken sponsoring activities around the James Bond film franchise.[13] Alcohol Change says, "The multi-channel nature of alcohol marketing means that the potential reach of drinks industry messages is potentially enormous. One particular concern is that alcohol marketing reaches many people well-below the legal drinking age, and studies have shown that children as young as 10 and 11 years are often very familiar with alcohol brands."[14]

---

[12] DavidH. Jernigan, *Alcohol marketing: Overview of the landscape*, Center on Alcohol Marketing and Youth Department of Health, Behavior and Society Johns Hopkins, Bloomberg School of Public Health https://cpb-us-e1.wpmucdn.com/sites.dartmouth.edu/dist/3/1128/files/2017/08/Jernigan_presentation.pdf [17.3.21]

[13] Nicholas Barber, *Does Bond's product placement go too far?*, BBC Culture https://www.bbc.com/culture/article/20151001-does-bonds-product-placement-go-too-far [17.3.21]

[14] *Making Sure Alcohol is Marketed Responsibly*, Alcohol Change UK. https://alcoholchange.org.uk/policy/policy-insights/making-sure-alcohol-is-marketed-responsibly [17.3.21]

I know of individuals that have experience of drinking because of advertising including a friend that watched an M&S TV advertisement featuring a glass of white wine lovingly poured into a glass, and promptly went out to buy a bottle of wine, ending three months of not drinking. The combination of huge spending on branding and marketing, government lobbying, traditional advertising, and the funding of independent groups that advise us to drink safely, has led to an increase in global consumption from 21 billion liters in 1990 to 35.7 billion liters in 2017 - an increase of 70%.[15] It is well known that men have historically drunk more than women, and they have suffered more harm. This isn't because alcohol works differently on men. Both sexes are equally susceptible to the effects of alcohol but alcohol marketing has traditionally leaned towards men via sports sponsorship for example. Now the major alcohol companies have figured out that they have an opportunity to make more money from growing the female customer base, and developing the future customer base by targeting children. Movendi International in its article *How Big Alcohol Converts Women to Alcohol*, says, "Women are one of Big Alcohol's major targets along with children and youth. There are various methods the industry uses to try and convert women into using alcohol."[16]

Media pressure

The media tend to present alcohol in a positive light by showing drinking as glamorous, and as a key part of characters' positive attributes. In a study by Joel W. Grube, he found, "Drinking was associated with wealth or luxury in 34 percent of films containing alcohol references," and "Portrayals of negative consequences of drinking are relatively rare. In all, 57 percent of films with alcohol references portrayed no consequences to the user. Similar findings have emerged from other content analyses. Thus, at least one lead character drank in 79 percent of the top money-making American films from 1985 to

---

[15] Jakob Manthey et al. *Global alcohol exposure between 1990 and 2017 and forecasts until 2030: a modelling study.* https://www.thelancet.com/journals/lancet/article/PIIS0140-6736(18)32744-2/ [17.3.21]

[16] *How Big Alcohol Converts Women to Alcohol*, Movendi International. https://movendi.ngo/news/2020/06/24/how-big-alcohol-converts-women-to-alcohol/ [17.3.21]

1995 ... [and] 96 percent of those films contained references supportive of alcohol use."[17]

It's no surprise that Hollywood represents drinking alcohol as a positive character attribute when the drinks industry spends large amounts of money on product placements in films, including films aimed at children. The American Academy of Pediatrics reported, "Alcohol brand placements in popular movies of all ratings nearly doubled during the past two decades... particularly in child-rated movies." James D. Sargent, MD, FAAP, a professor in the departments of Pediatrics and Community & Family Medicine at the Geisel School of Medicine at Dartmouth and an author of the study added "For alcohol companies, when a favorite star uses a certain brand of alcohol, that brand gets linked to all the characteristics young admirers see in their movie idol. That's why it's no surprise that the brands commonly shown in movies are the most highly advertised brands, and the same brands underage drinkers tend to drink."[18]

We see male lead characters in films drinking alcohol as part of their lifestyle and as part of the development of the story, where it is designed to show how resilient or masculine they are, and where being drunk never seems to interfere with the character's methods. Detectives, members of police forces and criminals with big plans are often shown drinking as part of their investigative work or planning. In a number of criminal dramas focused on the drug trade, for example Breaking Bad and Queen of the South, drinking tequila is represented as a display of power or machismo, with criminal bosses downing large measures of the drink, seemingly with no negative effects. I know from experience that if I am trying to get things done, a beer or glass

---

[17] Joel W. Grube, *Alcohol in the Media: Drinking Portrayals, Alcohol Advertising, and Alcohol Consumption Among Youth, Reducing Underage Drinking, A Collective Responsibility*, ed. Richard J Bonnie et al. https://www.ncbi.nlm.nih.gov/books/NBK37586/ [17.3.21]

[18] Samantha Cukier, James D. Sargent, *Trends in alcohol brand placements in top U.S. Movies, 1996-2015*, American Academy of Pediatrics. https://www.eurekalert.org/pub_releases/2017-05/aaop-amio42617.php [17.3.21]

of wine would get in the way and cause me to lose focus, and a large shot of tequila would seriously interfere with my plans.

There are portrayals of problem drinkers in the movies and in some rare cases drinking is shown in a particularly negative light, for example in Flight, the 2012 film that features Denzel Washington as a pilot, who drinks heavily, but more often films include positive outcomes for problem drinkers. The unlikely message being that lead characters deliver a positive result despite their drinking. In 1982's The Verdict, Paul Newman plays a lawyer who is given a chance to prosecute a big medical negligence case when a client turns up out of the blue. The lead character is drinking heavily every day but wins the case despite the drinking. Happy was a 2017 TV series about a heavy drinking ex-police detective successfully solving a child kidnapping case against the odds. These are typical of films that allow us to believe that individuals can achieve big things despite consuming alcohol, but the fact of the matter is that heavy drinkers will generally be less functional, and their alcohol consumption will tend to interfere in their work, relationships and their personal lives.

In popular music alcohol is part of the mythologising of wealth and status with Courvoisier and Cristal champagne namechecked in hip hop tracks and a tendency to present expensive alcoholic drinks as part of the bling and conspicuous consumption that is typical of the genre. Being tipsy and drunk is seen as sexy and fun in pop music lyrics, and often music videos are shot in bars and clubs that provide a positive sense that the drinking environment is a place of excitement and good taste. The Alcohol Rehab Guide says, "Themes of alcohol use were most apparent in rap and hip-hop music. These genres accounted for 37.7% of the songs that mentioned alcohol, and most frequently referenced tequila, vodka, cognac, and champagne. Country music was the second most alcohol-prevalent genre, with 32% of the mentions being found in country songs. Third was pop music, which accounted for 30.5% of the mentions. Unlike rap and hip-hop, country and pop music most typically referenced whiskey and beer. The study also found that songs in all of these genres widely portrayed alcohol in a positive light, and rarely presented the negative consequences associated with alcohol use."[19] It continues: "Pop culture plays a significant role in people's lives. According to the Social Learning Model, people learn not only by direct experience but also by exposure to modeled behavior, such as that represented in popular music. Individuals that are exposed to representations of drinking and alcohol use are more likely to engage in those behaviors themselves if they are represented in a positive light and associated with desirable affluences."[20]

Peer pressure

As well as the pressure of the media and marketing by the drinks industry every drinker knows that the most powerful advocates for consuming alcohol are their fellow drinkers. Drinkers need to recruit new people to join them in their consumption of alcohol so they pressure the people around them to drink. The peer pressure is so powerful, I know individuals who feel they can't go to a pub or restaurant and refuse to drink, because the people they know put so much pressure on them. Non drinkers can go to the pub with 100% certainty that they don't want to consume alcohol. But the occasional drinker, or a drinker that is trying to drink less is going to get the hard sell from their drinking friends. Non drinkers, once they have made certain that they don't drink will often hear the same thing from drinkers: "You don't drink? Good for you. I wish I didn't drink."

Who convinced us to have our first drink? Other drinkers. When we weren't sure, and we wavered, or when we were determined not to drink, who convinced us that we were wrong and made sure we had a drink in our hand? Other drinkers. Nature has given us a set of controls and warning signs that told us when we started drinking that alcohol was poisonous to us, and these same signals remind us, via hangovers and anxiety, that alcohol has a negative effect every time we drink. Yet we still bow to peer pressure and allow other

---

[19] Jena Hilliard, *Alcohol in Music,* Alcohol Rehab Guide, https://www.alcoholrehabguide.org/alcohol/alcohol-in-popular-culture/alcohol-in-music/ [17.3.21]

[20] *Alcohol in Music*

drinkers to dictate our alcohol intake. We've all experienced trying to leave the pub and being told by a friend that we have to have one more. The system of buying rounds for each other also causes pressure. Four people drinking together are likely to drink four pints or glasses of wine each, or if they are on a bender, eight each, because the round system of drink buying is so ingrained. We can't leave without buying a round for the group.

7

Alcohol and sleep

Humans need around seven or eight hours sleep a night to give us much needed mental and physical recovery.[21] We have two sleeping states, deep sleep and REM sleep. Our deep sleep sees increased blood flow delivering oxygen, nutrients and growth hormones to aid physical recovery,[22] so it is no surprise that vigorous exercise results in more deep sleep. REM means rapid eye movement and refers to the sleeping state when we dream, process memories and this is when our physical state most resembles our waking state. Research suggests that REM sleep is key to mental recovery and there are links between mental illness and poor sleep, showing that lack of good sleep may exacerbate or cause mental illness. The Mental Health Foundation says, "Sleep is as important to our health as eating, drinking and breathing. It allows our bodies to repair themselves and our brains to consolidate our memories and process information... Poor sleep is linked to physical problems such as a weakened immune system and mental health problems such as

---

[21] *Sleep and mental health*, Harvard Medical School.   https://www.health.harvard.edu/ newsletter_article/sleep-and-mental-health [17.3.21]

[22] John Delucchi, *Sleep: The Secret Ingredient of Injury Recovery*, Ortho Carolina. https://www.orthocarolina.com/media/sleep-the-secret-ingredient-of-injury-recovery [17.3.21]

anxiety and depression."[23]

In sleep nature has given us an amazing tool for physical and mental recovery. We each have a system for fixing our injuries, healing our bruises, fighting off diseases, and ensuring our rational mind works as it should. Sleep is key to the development and maintenance of almost all animals, us included. During the day we make use of our mental and physical abilities to complete tasks, work and play, and the stresses, strains and injuries that we suffer are resolved and repaired during our sleep. Whenever we are ill, or have suffered an injury, we are told to rest and get lots of sleep because this is the time that our body works to fight off infection and make repairs to ensure we heal. Again, this is an example of our natural system working to protect us and keep us in tip top condition.

If we go to bed with alcohol in our system our natural sleep patterns are impacted. Even small amounts of alcohol cause our REM sleep to be disturbed. When a drinker goes to bed with alcohol in his or her system they will typically enter a much longer deep sleep that lasts about five hours followed by a period of restless sleep which continues until the drinker is fully awake. The Sleep Foundation says, "Drinking alcohol before bed can add to the suppression of REM sleep during the first two cycles."[24] The extended deep sleep prevents the drinker experiencing the REM sleep needed for mental recovery. The result of sleeping with alcohol in the system is waking up feeling tired, and hungover drinkers will often feel this effect, even after having slept for seven or eight hours.

Having too much deep sleep doesn't sound like a problem but if it is at the expense of REM sleep, the sleep that is essential for mental recovery, then the

---

[23] Dr. Dan Robotham et al. *Sleep Matters, The impact of sleep on health and wellbeing,* Mental Health Foundation. https://www.mentalhealth.org.uk/publications/sleep-report [17.3.21]

[24] Danielle Pacheco, *Alcohol and Sleep,* Sleep Foundation. https://www.sleepfoundation.org/nutrition/alcohol-and-sleep [17.3.21]

result of alcohol infused sleep will lead to less than perfect cognitive ability. Good sleep is extremely important to mental wellbeing, and interrupting nature's mechanism for keeping us mentally sound isn't ideal. Drinkers that drink every day should expect their mental soundness to diminish due to regular alcohol disturbed sleep.

There is a secondary impact on our sleeping as the result of drinking and that is the high levels of stress hormones that stay in the system after drinking. For the occasional drinker the levels of cortisol, produced as a reaction to consuming alcohol, are low and may not interrupt sleep. Heavy drinkers though, both binge drinkers and daily drinkers, will have raised levels of cortisol in their system and this can lead to insomnia and poor sleep. I know a number of heavy drinkers that have suffered from insomnia and have turned to sleeping pills to help them sleep. Remember that in our natural state, free of alcohol, free of stresses and worry, we should all sleep fitfully and fully. It is obviously beneficial for any drinker, and especially heavy drinkers, to stop drinking and rediscover healthy normal sleep.

Tiredness is nature's way of getting us to sleep, because we need to recover. Our amazing system of controls that works to keep us safe tells us we are tired so that we either go to bed for a night's sleep, or take a nap. A drinker that consumed too much the night before will feel tired all day and for good reason. Last night's sleep was interrupted by the alcohol in the drinker's system and they didn't get a good night's sleep. The drinker's body and mind needs rest, and the signals are clear - get some sleep! But the drinker's fellow drinkers will do their best to persuade the drinker to go to the pub. "I'm tired," the drinker will say, "I should go home." but the fellow drinkers will say, "come to the pub for one drink." and here is where the dangerous properties of alcohol will negatively impact the drinker's system and controls. The first alcoholic drink interferes with the safety mechanism that is trying to get the drinker to go home to get some sleep. As soon as the drinker has consumed the first drink they suddenly won't feel tired any more. The brain now fails to signal tiredness because the system has been anesthetised, and flooded again with cortisol, the stress chemical that the body produces to counter the anesthetic. The drinker's judgement has been affected by the alcohol. The first glass will also cause the drinker to want to drink again, and the tiredness will be relegated even further. At this point the drinker is doomed to another night of consumption. Alcohol has negatively impacted nature's efforts to keep the individual safe.

8

Social life and alcohol

It is difficult to imagine a social life without alcohol when it appears to play such a key part of the way we interact with each other. Our culture is so infused with alcohol that it seems we can't socialise without drinking, can't enjoy a nice meal without consuming alcohol, can't celebrate without booze. It is generally accepted that drinking is a necessary part of the social experience. We can't believe that a social event can function without drinking. Imagine a wedding invite that specifies no alcohol will be available. There'd be outrage!

We are social creatures by nature and although it seems that alcohol is a key part of our interaction, because it is so ingrained in our culture, in fact drinking is detrimental to our social interaction. It interferes with our emotional control, our ability to communicate and our judgement. In small doses it affects our conversation, our sense of humour and our ability to do what we do best - socialise with our fellow humans. In moderate doses we become unstable, overly loud, sweaty and obnoxious, and when we consume large doses we become incoherent and out of control.

Our social tendencies keep us alive longer. A number of studies have shown that humans that are more social tend to be happier and live longer. The

Roseto effect (from a study of the town of Roseto)[25] shows that close social groupings result in less heart disease and longer lives, and there are a number of studies that show that loneliness causes a variety of conditions that shorten lifespan. The residents of Okinawa Japan, who live longer than anyone else on earth, have powerful social networks to support people well into old age and this aspect of their lives leads to low incidences of heart disease, cancer and dementia[26].

We have been engineered by nature to mingle with each other. Our natural social tendencies allow us to make friends, and maintain those friendships, find partners for sex in order to reproduce, to find a partner for life to keep us secure and to engage in competitive interactions to allow us to establish a social order. Like monkeys, or other animals that live in packs, we perform better in groups where historically we have been more secure and well protected, more able to complete tasks using complementary abilities, and more able to stay alive. It's no wonder then that nature rewards us for being social and interacting successfully with one another.

Think of a typical social event where people get together in a group. At first each attendee is naturally shy and a little wary but as they start to mingle, they relax and share more of themselves. This shyness is natural and normal and we all feel it, even people who appear outwardly confident. Our individual shyness soon dissipates in a social setting and we find ourselves laughing and smiling with each other. We tell stories and jokes as we compete with each other and flirt with the opposite sex. As we relax and begin to enjoy ourselves we feel the effect of the positive chemicals that are the result of our social interaction. Our system provides us with hormones that make us feel

---

[25] Joel Khan, The Roseto Effect: The Amazing Power of Relationships for Heart Health, Thrive Global, https://medium.com/thrive-global/the-roseto-effect-the-amazing-power-of-relationships-for-heart-health-ffdd49b77624 [17.3.21]

[26] Okinawa, Japan Secrets of the world's longest-living women

good, oxytocin and dopamine,[27] the natural reward that nature provides to us for being good social creatures. We become relaxed, happy, content and glowing with the experience of interaction. This is the natural, normal social experience and it is central to every human.

To see this in effect spend some time at a children's party. The kids arrive shy and nervous, worrying that they don't know anyone but within minutes are laughing, having fun and running around together without a care in the world. The happy hormones that nature provides cause the kids to be energetic, fun and carefree. We tend to mistake this natural effect as the result of the kids intake and for this reason there is a myth that fizzy drinks and sugar cause a behaviour change in children, causing them to run riot.

The key mistake drinkers make is to confuse the positive feelings of social interaction with the alcohol that they consumed. Every drinker will be able to look back to a perfect moment at a party when the vibe was just right. The music, the people, the setting, all converged into a powerful moment that lodged in the memory. And that memory will include the consumption of alcohol. Every time a drinker feels the amazing happy buzz of a great social situation, they will have associated that with the alcohol: What a great party, and I remember the amazing wine I was drinking. Yes, the event was amazing, but luckily the drinker hadn't drunk too much of the alcohol for it to ruin the evening. Parties work perfectly well without the alcohol and the happy hormones of successful social interaction will provide the warm happy glow. It wasn't the wine that gave the drinker the buzz at the party, it was the natural interaction with the other party guests.

The second mistake drinkers make is to believe that a drink relieves the natural feeling of shyness. Shyness is a normal part of our interaction with our fellow

---

[27] Node Smith, *Oxytocin and Dopamine: The Rewards of Socializing*, Naturopathic News. https://ndnr.com/naturopathic-news/oxytocin-and-dopamine-the-rewards-of-sociability/ [17.3.21]

humans and it prevents us from making a fool of ourselves, ensuring that we fit into a new social grouping. Although drinkers tell themselves that they'll feel less shy after a drink, drinking alcohol does not make us less shy. Because it is an anesthetic it numbs our natural senses and interferes with our natural social instincts. When we drink we lose our natural inhibitions which are in place for a good reason. Within a glass of wine or two drinkers will have quickly moved from the shy stage to being less good at conversation, repetitive, poor listeners, less empathetic to others, less funny, less good at controlling emotions. In short drinkers believe that a drink makes them less shy but the alcohol quickly causes drinkers to become exactly what they shouldn't be in a social situation - loud, obnoxious, boring and overbearing. Alcohol doesn't make the people that consume it more confident. In fact it interferes with the natural need to exert self control, to be an appropriately behaved member of the social group.

Non-drinkers go to the pub to see friends, to meet new people, to have fun, to find out what friends have been doing, and to enjoy the banter and laughs. Like everybody, they are shy when they arrive but they will quickly warm up and enjoy the situation, without an alcoholic drink in hand. Everybody likes the social aspect of a night in the pub but as the drinkers in the pub consume more alcohol they become more drunk and more annoying. The non-drinker will tend to leave at a sensible time and go home to bed for a good night's sleep. Non-drinkers see the effect of alcohol on the drinkers they socialise with - they become less funny, less bright and less good at conversation starting with drink number one, and progressively getting worse as they drink more.

Imagine being the only drinker at a social event where nobody else is drinking. As the only drinker there you would notice immediately that your stories are boring to the people around you, that you have become less funny and more repetitive, and you may become angry, tearful or overly joyous as the alcohol causes you to lose control of your emotions. The only drinker at a dry event would stand out, and his or her behaviour would be considered annoying and anti-social. It's ironic to note that the alcohol that we consider to be core to our social interaction would result in anti-social behaviour if a drinker continued to consume it.

The reverse experience is further evidence of the negative effects of alcohol. Spend the night sober while the people around you at the party or in the pub drink themselves into a state. Will you see shy people becoming more confident? No but you will see interesting, bright people with great personalities becoming more dull, more repetitive and less controlled. The tears, the unchecked emotions, the arguments and the fight outside the pub later are proof that alcohol is detrimental to the social interaction.

One of the big misunderstandings about alcohol that is repeated by scientists, medical practitioners and drinkers is that it makes people feel good. It isn't actually a nice sensation. If a drinker tries drinking out of context they will see that it is an unpleasant experience. Drinking a shot of tequila before a meeting at work for example, or when the drinker is at the library trying to find a book. The actual experience of consuming alcohol isn't positive. Drinkers confuse the positive experience of social interaction with their consumption of alcohol and they mistake the positive buzz of the social interaction with the effect of the alcohol. Only when we decouple them can we see them for what they really are.

Pubs work because they are full of drinkers on the same trajectory. By and large everybody in the pub starts consuming alcohol at the same time, and most drinkers consume alcohol at the same rate. The rate at which alcohol is consumed is not a free choice, it is the result of the rate at which our bodies process the alcohol we have already drunk. At closing time the mass of punters leave the pub having spent the evening with a pub full of people that legitimize their behaviour by behaving in the same way. It appears to be OK to get progressively more pissed with a room full of people getting progressively more pissed.

Social interactions work very well without alcohol. A drinker that decides to stop drinking, and chooses to attend social events without consuming alcohol will see a number of related benefits. It can be a revelation for a drinker that decides to go out with friends and stay sober. It is fun, the experience is much cheaper, and the social interaction means the evening will be positive. An evening without alcohol means waking up feeling fresh and well rested the next morning, and there is minimal risk of embarrassing oneself in front of one's peers. Drinkers that believe they have to drink feel deprived and will not be able to enjoy the evening but this is just a mindset issue, and a simple change of belief is enough for an evening free of alcohol to be a great evening.

Further evidence of the social experience can be found in a muslim country such as Morocco or a dry state such as Tamil Nadu in India.[28] Social groupings in these places work perfectly well as friends and family members gather to chat, drink tea or coffee, laugh and gossip. These locations are not made up of millions of individuals deprived of alcohol. They interact perfectly well, forming relationships and thriving on their natural social abilities.

Our society includes the belief we need to drink to be able to socialise and that alcohol oils the wheels of social interaction. Again and again we see our peers negatively affected by alcohol and yet we hold onto these beliefs. The first drinking experience at a social event wasn't something natural. None of us entered our teenage years believing that we wouldn't be able to interact with people without an alcoholic drink in our hand. We all socialised in playgrounds, parks and parties as children. But the drinkers that convinced us to start drinking wanted us to believe otherwise. The people that told us we needed to drink at social events were other drinkers. The people that feel they can't manage a social event without a drink are the same people that need to recruit more people to join their ranks.

The belief that alcohol is necessary to social interaction is a little bit ridiculous.

---

[28] *Alcohol prohibition in Tamil Nadu,* Wikipedia. https://en.wikipedia.org/wiki/Alcohol_prohibition_in_Tamil_Nadu [17.3.21]

Kids don't need to consume alcohol to enjoy the parties they attend. When we were 10 years old we never refused to go to a party unless we could drink wine. We didn't drink a can of lager just so we could have a conversation with a stranger. As children, each of us was a bit shy, a bit uncertain of ourselves and we took time to warm to social situations. Nothing changes as adults, we're still the same. The alcohol is detrimental to our social interaction but we believe, wrongly, that we need it to mingle.

9

Emotional control

In daily life we are able to control and manage our emotions. Our emotions are a necessary part of our protection systems to keep us safe and allow us to function among other humans successfully. We need to feel upset, angry and frustrated in certain situations so that we take action or avoid those situations, but we typically bring our emotions under control very quickly. As an example imagine that you bump into a clumsy pedestrian on the pavement. You might feel a flush of anger and you may swear or mutter, but this flash of anger will quickly reside. An argument with your partner over a trivial matter is just that - trivial, and although we feel our emotional state quickly change from frustration to annoyance and to anger, we can quickly bring this under control. When we drink though the alcohol that we consume interferes with our ability to control these emotions, effectively blocking the off switch, so that once we become angry, tearful, upset or humiliated, we can't quickly revert to our normal calm state. The result of this is arguments that continue far longer than they should, fights between drinkers who would otherwise find a more natural way of resolving a dispute, fallouts between couples where a throwaway remark has led to tears and misery of despair that can't be switched off.

Imagine a situation where a participant requires a cool head, for example in a courtroom, a negotiation, or doing a business deal. To be a successful participant, to swing an outcome in our favour we all know how important it is to keep control of our emotions, and even small amounts of alcohol can have an impact on our ability to do this. Each of us has the capacity to be successful in social situations, in negotiations or in a meeting.

10

Memories

At the front of our brain is our new memory maker, the hippocampus.[29] It's a brilliant tool, turning our day to day experiences into a repository of memories that keep us safe from harm, allow us to consider our behavior and enable us to learn and develop. Humans are incredible creatures and our strength over other species is our ability to pass on knowledge and learning. An individual's memory of an event can be turned into a story for others that will allow him or her to teach their fellow humans so that if they encounter a similar situation, they will know what to do. This phenomenal part of the way our brain operates is something we take for granted and, like every aspect of our natural system, it is perfect.[30]

Alcohol's effect on the hippocampus is dramatic. When we drink enough, and the alcohol in blood content gets to a certain level (it depends on the drinker but double the UK drink drive limit seems to do the trick for many of us)[31] the hippocampus switches off and stops making new memories. The result of this

---

[29] Kendra Cherry, *What is the Hippocampus?* Very Well Mind, https://www.verywellmind.com/what-is-the-hippocampus-2795231 [17.3.21]

[30] *How Are Memories Formed?* Queensland Brain Institute, https://qbi.uq.edu.au/brain-basics/memory/how-are-memories-formed [17.3.21]

[31] Nicolle Monico, *Memory Loss, Blackouts, & Binge Drinking Dangers,* American Addiction Centers, https://www.alcohol.org/effects/blackouts-dangers/ [17.3.21]

is a blackout. We continue to operate, albeit very drunk, but our hippocampus does not record the events. At that point we are probably way past the point of any sensible judgement and our emotional control has switched off so our behaviour will be negatively affected. In the morning our friends have to talk us through the events of the evening before and fill in the gaps. At that point drinkers often don't believe how they acted and the stories of their behaviour sound as alien as if they weren't even there. There is a very real sense of being out of control at this point, and it can be very alarming to hear that we were acting seemingly without being aware of our actions. Alcohol exerts control over drinkers and being told about something we did, and that we have no knowledge of, is a great example of that loss of control. A blackout is evidence that at the time we needed to be most in control, when our alcohol intake was excessive, when we should have been taking care of ourselves we appeared to be on auto-pilot and totally irresponsible.

Rose Tinted Spectacles

Human memory is a fascinating thing. Our brains prioritise positive memories over negative ones. When we think back to holidays, social events, school days, etc we typically think of the positive aspects and our brain emphasises the good over the bad. Imagine if our brains did the opposite and only emphasised the negative - we would all be depressed and miserable. We wouldn't leave the house if we believed everything we'd ever done in the past had been bad in some way.

When we drink we often wake up the next morning feeling hungover, embarrassed or ashamed about our behaviour, sometimes with parts of the evening missing from our memory. We feel terrible, and we have the sensation of having been out of control the night before. At that point the drinker clearly remembers the negative aspects of the night before, and the negatives that are present right now - the lethargy, the discomfort, the headache, the anxiety, the dry mouth, etc. At that point we have all made a resolution to never drink again! But within a few days our memory of the previous nights drinking is so different. Our rose tinted spectacles have prioritised the positive aspects, and we now look back and say What a brilliant night we had! This useful trick that our brain plays on us causes us to forget the embarrassment and the discomfort, and we drink again, repeating the same pattern having forgotten the lessons we learned.

11

Confidence and fear

There is a common misconception that alcohol gives us confidence or reduces fear. Fear exists to keep us safe and stop us injuring or killing ourselves. We don't like going near a cliff edge or a burning building for good reason. Our natural system of controls keeps us safe by making us fearful of dangerous situations. And the stress we experience when we are forced into dangerous situations is our body's attempt to get us ready to flee - the fight or flight response. The adrenaline and cortisol that flood our system make us feel alert and on edge so that we can escape danger and deal with potential threats. Fear works to keep us out of dangerous situations and stops us being reckless. When we drink, the alcohol interferes with this very important safety mechanism and we become less aware of the potential for injury. Most us us don't do stupid stunts, climb lampposts or attempt daring feats when we are sober but these are the sort of things that drinkers have a go at after they have had a few drinks. Obviously if any of us ever decide to attempt a risky ambitious stunt we generally make sure that we are stone cold sober. Do we fancy going rock climbing, hang-gliding or skiing? Lets get drunk first, said nobody ever. The Accident and Emergency ward on a Friday night is full of individuals who have suffered head injuries or other mishaps because they have failed to listen to their instinctive capacity for safety and wellbeing.

It shouldn't be a surprise that alcohol is a factor in a number of suicides. The conscious desire of the individual to end their own life will be at odds with the natural instinct for survival. Any human that moves a blade towards an artery or approaches a cliff edge or wraps a rope around their neck will instinctively feel fear, and may find it difficult to do what they set out to do. Because alcohol clouds our judgement and reduces our natural instincts for safety, drinking before a suicide attempt will interfere with the brain's natural protection systems, reducing natural levels of fear and increasing recklessness. In this New York Times article entitled *Alcohol a Common Factor in Suicides* a report found around a third of suicide victims had alcohol in their blood, and the Centers for Disease Control and Prevention reported that in a large sample of suicide victims, "one in four had been legally drunk, with a blood alcohol content at or above the federal standard." Dr. Alex Crosby, quoted in the article said, "It leads to disinhibition, and it can enhance feelings of hopelessness and depression. Alcohol impairs judgment and can lead to much more impulsive behavior."[32]

The picture is similar for crime. Most of us, through a combination of moral judgement, adherence to the law, and care for our fellow humans don't commit crime, or do each other harm. Alcohol interferes with our good judgement though and plays havoc with our ability to exercise restraint, at the same time that it interferes with our emotional control. The result is violence, impulsive actions that can cause harm, and reckless behaviour, leading to criminal acts that we wouldn't consider when we are sober. The US Bureau of Justice Statistics in its study *Alcohol and Crime*, found "Two-thirds of victims who suffered violence by an intimate (a current or former spouse, boyfriend, or girlfriend) reported that alcohol had been a factor. Among spouse victims, 3 out of 4 incidents were reported to have involved an offender who had been drinking. By contrast, an estimated 31% of stranger victimizations where the victim could determine the absence or presence of alcohol were perceived to be alcohol-related." and "Among the 5.3 million convicted offenders under

---

[32] Roni Caryn Rabin, *Alcohol a Common Factor in Suicides*, New York Times, https://www.nytimes.com/2009/06/19/health/19suicide.html [17.3.21]

the jurisdiction of corrections agencies in 1996, nearly 2 million, or about 36%, were estimated to have been drinking at the time of the offense. The vast majority, about 1.5 million, of these alcohol-involved offenders were sentenced to supervision in the community: 1.3 million on probation and more than 200,000 on parole."[33]

The New York Times also reported: "Illegal drugs and alcohol helped lead to the imprisonment of 4 out of 5 inmates in the [U.S.'s] prisons and jails, a three-year study has found... The report... by the National Center on Addiction and Substance Abuse at Columbia University, determined that of 1.7 million prisoners in 1996, 1.4 million had violated drug or alcohol laws, had been high when they committed their crimes, had stolen to support their habit or had a history of drug and alcohol abuse that led them to commit crimes."[34]

For most of us criminal acts don't cross our radar because our moral compass keeps us legal and safe. Alcohol interferes with our good judgement, and causes reckless and impulsive behaviour. For any career criminal, bank robber, drug dealer or member of an organised crime family that wants to stay out of prison it is worth remembering that to be professional it is best to be organised and well prepared when it comes to planning and carrying out crime. Consuming alcohol is likely to lead to impulsive and unplanned reckless behaviour, which in turn is likely to lead to arrest.

Confidence is an interesting aspect of human interaction. We look at each other and judge our fellow humans based on how confident they appear. Successful people seem super confident, but we all have confidence levels that rise and fall. Confidence increases when we are comfortable with our

---

[33] Lawrence A. Greenfeld, *Alcohol and Crime, An Analysis of National Data on the Prevalence of Alcohol Involvement in Crime*, US Department of Justice. https://www.bjs.gov/content/pub/pdf/ac.pdf [17.3.21]

[34] Christopher S Wren, *Drugs or Alcohol Linked to 80% of Inmates*, New York Times, https://www.nytimes.com/1998/01/09/us/drugs-or-alcohol-linked-to-80-of-inmates.html [17.3.21]

situation and surroundings, or when we are well prepared. We are all less confident in new surroundings, with new people and experiencing new events. Drinking alcohol is perceived to be a confidence booster and we talk of dutch courage, the confidence provided by consuming it. The origin of the phrase is rooted in conflict and refers to soldiers that were administered alcohol before attacking the enemy during the Anglo-Dutch conflict. Alcohol is likely to be beneficial to an attack because it reduces the fear that we would naturally feel, and this reduced fear makes us more reckless. We have all seen the effects of alcohol on individuals who would normally resolve conflicts calmly and sensibly without resorting to violence, who after a few drinks seem quick to fight each other without restraint.

For those of us who feel less confident in social situations than we would like to, alcohol will make individuals less sensitive to the worry of social mixing by interfering with the useful and natural levels of fear, but it does not make anybody more confident. For someone who always drinks at social events, making a change, and deciding not to drink, will build confidence once the individual has tackled a social event without the crutch of alcohol. We all become more confident as we successfully socialise, chat to people and relax in the natural social environment. Drinkers that use alcohol to mitigate natural shyness will argue that there is a sweet spot when just the right amount of alcohol in their system makes them feel they are in control, the conversation seems to flow easily and the social interaction seems natural and normal. However, this sweet spot is just a moment in a long night of alcohol consumption and is typically followed by deteriorating social interaction as the detrimental alcohol takes effect.

Imagine the typical situations where we need to be confident, for example if we are put into a leadership position, or when we are pitching an idea, or presenting information, performing on stage, or we are on a date and want to impress our potential partner. At these moments confidence comes from preparation and experience. If we are well rehearsed, have practiced our pitch, know our lines or can successfully relay information then we ought to be confident. Having a drink may appear to calm the nerves before a stressful event but the alcohol will interfere with our abilities and will almost certainly create a situation where our performance deteriorates. There isn't a lot of difference between a social interaction and a business meeting or pitch. We go out dressed to impress and we need our bright mind and great social skills to persuade and convince our fellow humans that we should be liked, respected and fancied. At these moments we should avoid being unintentionally rude, boring, obnoxious and dull but this is what alcohol does to us. In the same way, in order to be a great partner on a date, staying sober will let our amazing personality shine.

12

Relaxation and stress

Drinkers mistakenly believe that drinking alcohol helps them to relax and to de-stress but in fact it does the opposite, and increases stress levels. The things that cause us stress are typically factors in our life that require us to take action, or to accept them. Stress at work is a good example and can be caused, for example, by a heavy workload, a change in working patterns or a demanding boss. The stress is recognisable and can be dealt with by putting in more hours, adapting to the new working pattern, and accepting that the demanding boss is a pain. Some stress is visible and easily identified, some requires professional help to identify.

Stress is another way that nature keeps us safe, and is a key part of our amazing system of controls. Our body and mind have to prioritise important things over less important things and stress is a signal to us that something is causing us pressure and needs resolving. If you are waking up in the middle of the night and turning things over in your mind it is because that thing is a priority and has the potential to cause harm. Stress is a normal part of our thinking but we should only be stressed temporarily, between the stressful scenario arising and subsequently being resolved.

Relaxation is the state of being calm and free of the things that are causing us stress. For example if we have a list of jobs that is causing us stress then getting those jobs done, and ticking things off our to do list, will make each of us more relaxed. If we can't relax because of something in our life that is out of our control such as a medical condition, trauma of some sort, or a situation that we can't change such as a death or divorce, then relaxation can generally be achieved by us accepting the situation, and this mirrors the typical guidance from counsellors - if we can't fix it we need to accept it.

Because alcohol is addictive, drinkers feel relief when they drink it, the relief being the satisfaction of the craving for alcohol. This relief can feel like a moment of relaxation. Drinkers have high levels of cortisol, the stress hormone in their system and this chemical causes them to feel edgy and anxious. An alcoholic drink anesthetises the drinker and provides relief from the anxiety. Alcohol does not have relaxing properties, it is an anesthetic that numbs the senses and reduces the capacity for feeling. Consuming alcohol feels relaxing when the anxious edgy feeling is temporarily relieved by the anesthetic effect of the alcohol. At the same time drinkers are likely to forget the stressful thing because the alcohol interferes with their judgement. The stressful thing requires our attention but when we drink alcohol we de-prioritise the stressful thing and cause our natural abilities to fail again.

Drinkers misunderstand alcohol as relaxing but this fallacy is also repeated by experts. Professor David Nutt, "world-renowned professor of neuropsy-chopharmacology, medical doctor and psychiatrist" (as he describes himself on the back cover of his recent book *Drink?)* is typical when he mistakenly says, "most people drink to relax," and of alcohol, "being both relaxing and pleasant to take..."[35] The Healthline website includes this similar, dubious statement in its article *Alcohol and Anxiety*: "At first, drinking can reduce fears and take your mind off of your troubles. It can help you feel less shy, give you a boost in mood, and make you feel generally relaxed."[36]

---

[35] David Nutt, *Drink?* Yellow Kite 2020

[36] *Alcohol and Anxiety*, Healthline, https://www.healthline.com/health/alcohol-and-anxiety# alcohol-effects [17.3.21]

Drinkers feel the anesthetic effect of alcohol as it calms the anxious feeling caused by the last drinks they had. Yesterday's drinks caused the drinker to feel anxious because of the stress chemical, cortisol that the body produced to counter the effect of the alcohol. The first drink of the day appears to relax the drinker but this is the effect of the anesthetic. The easiest way of testing the relaxing property of alcohol would be to give it to a non-drinker or a child and ask them if they feel relaxed after drinking it. A glass of wine appears to be relaxing to a drinker but a glass of wine would make a non-drinker or a child feel anesthetised, unsteady, out of control, and possibly make them sick. They would not describe the effect as relaxing.

If drinking alcohol was relaxing then we would expect the people who drink it the most to be the most relaxed. The opposite is true. People that consume a lot of alcohol tend to be on edge and anxious all the time. If drinking alcohol relieves stress then we would expect the biggest drinkers to have the least amount of stress in their lives. In fact we each think about everybody we know, we find that the individuals that are most stressed are also the ones that drink the most. People who drink alcohol tend to be less good at getting things done. The more drinkers consume, the less likely they are to tick off the things on their to do list. A solid session in the pub followed by a day of being hungover and lethargic takes about 24 hours out of the drinker's life and guarantees that he or she is not in a fit state to take any meaningful action during that time.

Drinking causes stress in two ways. It stops people from getting things done, so the thing that is causing stress on Friday is still there on Saturday, and because alcohol causes the body to produce cortisol, the stress hormone, it makes drinkers more anxious. The result of waking up with a hangover and feeling anxious is to make the stressful thing more stressful. The hungover drinker hasn't tackled the cause of the stress, now they are hungover and the anxiety is making the stress worse.

To be fully relaxed we shouldn't drink. Non-drinkers are naturally calm and able to deal with stress. Any individual with a lot to do, or experiencing a stressful situation, will find alcohol interferes with their ability to get those things done, and will make the stressful situation worse. Ambitious and driven individuals know that building a business, making sales, devising strategy, and creating an empire takes effort and discipline. For successful people relaxation and stress reduction come from achieving goals. These same people know that alcohol is highly detrimental and will interfere with their ability to perform well.

If an individual is experiencing a stressful day, alcohol will make it worse. Drinking will temporarily remove the stress because it is an anesthetic and will make the drinker temporarily forget about the thing that is causing the stress. But the cause is still there when the anesthetic wears off, and now the drinker has heightened anxiety exacerbating the situation. For any drinker that feels stressed the best decision they can make is to give up drinking. Within five days of the last drink a drinker will find that their anxiety levels will have reduced leaving them feeling calm. The extra time that a drinker frees up from not being in the pub or drinking at home, the increased energy levels that are the result of a good night's sleep, and having no hangover, will allow the non-drinker to charge through his or her to do list, ticking off the jobs that they have been putting off for years.

13

The effects of drinking

We use the word intoxicated for good reason to describe being drunk. Alcohol is toxic. There are other common terms to describe being drunk: legless, battered, hammered, wasted. These terms are not positive. As we move from first drink to second to third drink and beyond we introduce more alcohol into our system via the bloodstream and this has a significant effect on our brain and body. Here are some bullets showing alcohol content in blood (per 100ml) and the effect it has on our system:

- Alcohol content below 50mg: Some impairment in motor coordination and thinking ability

- Alcohol content between 50mg and 150mg: impaired concentration and judgement

- Alcohol content between 150 and 250mg: slurred speech, unsteady walking, nausea, double vision

- Alcohol content between 250 and 400mg: unresponsive/extremely drowsy; speech incoherent/confused; memory loss; vomiting

· Alcohol content over 400mg: breathing slowed, shallow or stopped; coma; death[37]

Even at minor concentrations the effect is described as an "impairment". Is it good to be impaired in any way? No, we should be operating at our best 100% of the time, as nature intended us to. Does our impaired concentration and judgement make us better? More social? Funnier? No, it makes us less good at listening to our friends, less good at the subtleties of conversation, less aware of our own need for restraint, more argumentative, more repetitive and more boring. If we keep drinking we move into the realm of physical deterioration and we slur our speech, we may have trouble walking, to the point where injuries could result from falling, and we can't see straight. This is a powerful and nasty poison but we willingly consume it night after night.

More than 250mg of alcohol in the blood causes the drinker to move into more dangerous territory. Being "unresponsive" is bad, vomiting (because the body recognises that the alcohol is a poison and is trying to keep the drinker safe), is bad and if the drinker has managed to get enough alcohol into his or her system death isn't far away. To be clear about the amounts in the table above, 250mg is roughly one tenth of half a teaspoon, or a bit more than a raindrop.

Here's a heartbreaking quote from a story of what happened when a 17 year old girl drank enough vodka to kill herself one evening, from a news feature entitled *15 Shots of Vodka Killed Our Daughter*:

> *When Shelby began to feel sick, Jane led her to the nearest bathroom to vomit. When Shelby seemed to pass out, she was propped against the*

---

[37] Brust, J. C. M. (2005). *Alcoholism*, In L. P. Rowland (Ed.), *Merritt's neurology* (11th ed.). Philadelphia: Lippincott Williams and Wilkins. Quoted in *Blood alcohol levels*, Alcohol.org.nz, https://www.alcohol.org.nz/alcohol-its-effects/about-alcohol/blood-alcohol-levels [17.3.21]

toilet for the night. Her young pal then left to be with Alyssa, who at this point was also sick from drinking, and periodically checked on Shelby. Clearly, this party had gone out of control.

[a friend] went to check on her and was horrified by what she found: Shelby was still slumped in the downstairs bathroom, completely motionless. Her head hung over the edge of the toilet bowl, her lip split from having slammed against the porcelain in a bout of violent heaving. Pulling Shelby up, Alyssa saw her friend's face streaked in blood. She tried to rouse her, but Shelby remained unresponsive. An older sister was summoned and phoned her father. He quickly returned to the house and dialed 911 to have an ambulance sent to his home right away because he'd found "a child that's here, and I don't think she's breathing." When asked if he was sure she wasn't breathing, he responded, "I can't ... I'm not sure she's alive right now."

Dispatchers instructed him on how to perform CPR, urging him to continue until medical help arrived. The EMTs who arrived on the scene found a weak pulse, but were unable to revive the girl. Shelby Allen was pronounced dead at 9:40 on the morning of December 20. Her blood-alcohol content was... four times the legal driving limit for adults in California.[38]

Obviously death is very rare. Most of us drink small amounts believing that it is harmless. Because alcohol is addictive though, one drink is very likely to lead to more drinks and because of this drinkers need to exercise restraint to say no, hopefully before they reach the more detrimental phases. Drinkers believe they are improved in some way under the influence of moderate amounts of alcohol and never plan to move into the high risk stages. Nobody goes to the pub or the party planning to be impaired, incoherent, or unresponsive but this sometimes happens. Drinkers accept that the risk of drinking is sometimes to

---

[38] Andrea Todd, *15 Shots of Vodka Killed Our Daughter*, Good Housekeeping, https://www.goodhousekeeping.com/life/parenting/a13054/binge-drinking-killed-shelby-allen/ [17.3.21]

fail to exercise restraint and to lose further control. The tradeoff is that they believe there are benefits to drinking and feel they cannot socialise without it.

The simple fact is that alcohol does not improve the mood of a non-drinker. It does not lift the spirits of non-drinkers. It is not relaxing to non-drinkers. It only works on drinkers and this is because it is addictive. A panel of non-drinkers made up of a cross-section of the population, young and old, in a laboratory setting would describe alcohol as an unpleasant anesthetic. They would tell you that the foul tasting liquid made them unsteady, clouded their thinking, made them lose their coordination and made them feel worse than they felt before they consumed it. They would not feel relaxed, euphoric or derive any pleasure from the experience.

There is an interesting effect that drinkers report when drinking and that is the improvement in the mood as they take the first sip. "Ah, that's better," coupled with an immediate sense of relaxation. Alcohol takes around five to 10 minutes to reach the brain but the mood of the drinker is improved immediately. This sense of relief, an improvement in mood caused by the administration of an addictive drug that has not yet had time to work, is evidence of the fallacy of drinking.[39] Alcohol appears to improve the mood of drinkers, feels relaxing to them, and makes them believe the experience is pleasurable because when they consume it they feel relief. They believe they need alcohol to socialise, and they associate good times with alcohol. It only works in context. In truth the effects of drinking are not pleasurable but the time in the pub is positive, as all social experiences should be. Alcohol on its own is not pleasurable, it is an unpleasant anesthetic that adversely affects us. Try a couple of vodkas for breakfast, or give the same vodka to a non-drinker or a child and they will tell you that it is not a pleasant experience.

The idea of alcohol as a mood improver or as a substance that makes drinkers

---

[39] *How Alcohol Impacts the Brain*, Northwestern Medicine, https://www.nm.org/healthbeat/healthy-tips/alcohol-and-the-brain [17.3.21]

feel good is repeated by the media and health practitioners as a reason why we consume alcohol. "Drinking alcohol can make humans feel pretty good, at least in the short term," from the BBC article *The science of alcohol: How booze affects your body* [40] and "It doesn't help that drinking, for a hot minute, makes you feel better,"[41] are typical quotes but alcohol only makes drinkers feel better and would not work on non-drinkers. Because drinkers have high levels of stress hormones in their system, they feel anxious and edgy. The next alcoholic drink has an anesthetic effect and provides relief. Alcohol as a pleasurable experience is a common belief but again is a biased view repeated and reinforced by drinkers.

---

[40] *The science of alcohol: How booze affects your body*, BBC Newsbeat, https://www.bbc.co.uk/news/newsbeat-30350860 [17.3.21]

[41] Meghan Rabbitt, Paul Schrodt, *8 Things That Happen When You Stop Drinking Alcohol*, Men's Health, https://www.menshealth.com/health/a19532341/what-happens-when-you-stop-drinking-alcohol/ [17.3.21]

14

Harms

In the 18th century it was common in England for children to be employed as chimney sweeps. Long before the law changed to make education mandatory, small boys were employed to do the dirty job of clambering into and up chimneys where they got incredibly dirty due to working in sooty conditions. Soot, the by-product of burning coal, became lodged in the difficult to reach parts of the body, and in an era where hygiene was not a priority, the presence of sooty skin caused cancers to develop, particularly testicular cancer. "chimney-sweep cancer was predominantly found in English chimney sweeps, probably because the chimney flues were narrower and Londoners often hired young boys aged between 4 and 7 years who could fit through the ducts."[42] The medical condition had an obvious cause - the residue of coal applied to the skin for an extended period of time caused cancer.

Coal smoke is not natural to humans, we have been reared in the outdoors and we have evolved to breathe clean air. It's no surprise that coal smoke and the residue of burnt carbon causes us harm. A topical poisonous chemical,

---

[42] Nadia Benmoussa et al. *Chimney-sweeps' cancer—early proof of environmentally driven tumourigenicity,* The Lancet, https://www.thelancet.com/journals/lanonc/article/PIIS1470-2045(19)30106-8/ [17.3.21]

meaning a poison that is applied to an area of the body, can cause cancers to develop in the location it is applied. If we breathe smoke the same carbon particles can cause us severe harm. During the 18th century England's cities burnt massive quantities of coal for heat and energy to the extent that entire cities were engulfed in toxic smoke. The harm to residents' health was dramatic. Over time legislation and regulation have reduced the toxicity of the air we breathe by reducing smoke in the atmosphere, but this work is still ongoing. In 2020 the Government is legislating against certain fuels that are burnt at home in fireplaces and stoves with the BBC reporting that, "The government said wood burning stoves and coal fires are the largest source of fine particulate matter (PM2.5), small particles of air pollution which find their way into the body's lungs and blood. Particulate matter is one of several pollutants caused by industrial, domestic and traffic sources."[43] The smoking ban that ensured that our public spaces were free of harmful tobacco smoke was finally introduced in 2007.

Coal smoke contains a range of dangerous chemicals[44] that are poisonous to humans in many ways. As a topical poison, coal residue causes cancer to develop on the skin. When it is inhaled it causes respiratory problems in the lungs and it can lead to lung cancer and other health problems.[45] Coal smoke is not something we should be around and when we are exposed to it we see increased health problems and death.[46] It is a substance that is not part of our natural environment and is obviously detrimental to us. The need for

---

[43] *Wood burners: Most polluting fuels to be banned in the home*, BBC News, https://www.bbc.co.uk/news/uk-51581817 [17.3.21]

[44] *Coal and Air Pollution*, Union of Concerned Scientists, https://www.ucsusa.org/resources/coal-and-air-pollution [17.3.21]

[45] *Indoor Emissions from the Household Combustion of Coal*, National Cancer Institute at the National Institutes of Health, https://www.cancer.gov/about-cancer/causes-prevention/risk/substances/indoor-coal [17.3.21]

[46] *Cooking with wood or coal is linked to increased risk of respiratory illness and death*, American Thoracic Society, quoted in Science Daily, https://www.sciencedaily.com/releases/2018/09/180921092447.htm [17.3.21]

energy has caused, and still causes, pollution to our natural environment which has the potential to harm us. The individuals that end up being harmed by coal smoke often are often not in a position to exercise free will to leave the polluted environment.

Like coal smoke, ethanol, the alcohol that is in our drinks, is a harmful poisonous substance that is foreign to our natural body. Like the coal soot and smoke, it causes topical harm in the area it is applied, and causes us harm when we consume it, both immediately and in the long term. It is a highly effective poison, produced through the natural process of fruit or grain rotting. It is naturally occurring but it is not natural for us to consume it. The smell and taste of it should put us off. We have evolved to reject things that taste and smell acrid and unpleasant. Like smoke which causes us to cough, alcohol smells nasty and tastes foul. If we had to drink it neat we would find it tastes disgusting and we would vomit it out immediately. Unlike coal smoke which affected those unlucky enough to live in an area where coal was burned, we are each free to choose whether or not we consume alcohol.

Here is an overview of ethanol from ChemicalSafetyFacts.org:

> "Ethanol is a common ingredient in many cosmetics and beauty products. It acts as an astringent to help clean skin, as a preservative in lotions and to help ensure that lotion ingredients do not separate, and it helps hairspray adhere to hair... Because ethanol is effective in killing microorganisms like bacteria, fungi and viruses, it is a common ingredient in many hand sanitizers... More than 97 percent of U.S. gasoline contains ethanol, typically in a mixture called E10, made up of 10 percent ethanol and 90 percent gasoline, to oxygenate the fuel and reduce air pollution. Ethanol has a higher octane number than gasoline, providing premium blending properties, according to the U.S. Department of Energy. Minimum octane number requirements prevent engine knocking and maintain drivability... Ethanol is highly flammable

and should not be used near open flames."[47]

A substance that is described as highly flammable, that kills microorganisms and that powers car engines doesn't sound like something we should voluntarily drink, and it is not surprising that something so alien to us will have detrimental effects.

Harms – Cancers

We process alcohol by using the equipment that nature provided to us to digest food. Drinkers consume alcohol by pouring it into the mouth where it travels down the throat, through the gut and out of the rectum. The liver processes it in an attempt to remove the dangerous chemical from our bodies. In the same way that coal dust and soot applied to the testicles of England's chimney sweeps caused cancers it shouldn't be a surprise to find that alcohol causes cancers of the mouth, throat, voice box (larynx), esophagus, colon and rectum, as well as, obviously, the organ that works hard to remove it from our bodies, the liver. It doesn't matter if the alcohol is in a 99p can of super strength cider, or a £1,000 bottle of rare vintage wine, the carcinogenic property is the same. Ethanol causes cancer and it causes cancer in the parts of our bodies where it travels.

Listerine is a mouthwash with high alcohol content. The bright sparks at Listerine that created the product decided to include a lot of alcohol to kill germs and it is marketed as a surefire way to control bad breath. Humans in their natural state, hydrated and eating the correct food shouldn't have bad breath. Listerine is an example of a product that is designed to solve a problem that nature has already solved. If any of us have bad breath we should change what we consume to revert to a natural state and our bad breath should go away. We don't need to wash our mouth with alcohol.

---

[47] *Ethanol (Ethyl Alcohol)*, Chemical Safety Facts.org, https://www.chemicalsafetyfacts.org/ethanol/ [17.3.21]

The alcohol content in the mouthwash administered to the mouth has been cited as causing cancer in the mouths of its users. I should point out that Listerine states, "No, LISTERINE® does not cause oral cancer. Scientists have compiled an extensive body of clinical data that has found no evidence or correlation between alcohol-based mouthwashes, such as LISTERINE® and oral cancer, including seven original studies and four reviews."[48] However the law firm, Parker Waichman LLP, that took legal action against Listerine said, "The Australian study, which involved 3,210 people, found daily mouthwash use was a 'significant risk factor' for oral cancer... The scientists found evidence that the ethanol in high-alcohol mouthwash increases the permeability of the mucosa to cancer-causing substances like nicotine. The toxic breakdown product of alcohol called acetaldehyde is also a carcinogen, and may accumulate in the oral cavity when swished around the mouth."[49] The World Dental Federation reporting on the Lancet's *Alcohol use and burden for 195 countries* study writes, "The *Lancet* study [about alcohol consumption] is particularly relevant to oral health, as it links alcohol use to four types of oral cancer: oesophageal cancer, larynx cancer, lip and oral cavity cancer, and pharynx and nasopharynx cancer. The study indicates that any level of alcohol consumption, even one drink per day, increases the relative risk of developing each of these cancers."[50]

We don't need a scientific background or medical training to see what is obvious to us. It is not natural to willingly administer a dangerous chemical to our bodies, and we shouldn't be surprised when that same chemical, travelling through the perfect and amazing equipment that we each have for ensuring that we are well nourished, subsequently causes harm. Cancers have the

---

[48] *Does LISTERINE® Cause Oral Cancer?*, https://www.listerine.com.au/does-listerine-cause-oral-cancer [17.3.21]

[49] *Listerine Mouthwash Lawsuit, Oral Cancer Side Effect, High Alcohol Mouthwash*, Parker Waichman LLP, Your Lawyer, https://www.yourlawyer.com/lawsuits/listerine/ [17.3.21]

[50] *Lancet report ties alcohol use to oral cancer – even moderate consumption is not without risk*, World Dental Federation, https://www.fdiworlddental.org/pt/news/20181011/lancet-report-ties-alcohol-use-to-oral-cancer-even-moderate-consumption-is-not-without-risk [17.3.21]

potential to kill us, and they tend to spread if they are not treated. Breast cancer risk also increases as alcohol intake rises, with Breast Cancer Now saying in clear language, "Regularly drinking alcohol increases your risk of developing breast cancer. The more you drink, the greater your risk."[51]

For the drinker that wants to know if their current level of alcohol consumption can cause cancer the answer is yes. Alcohol is carcinogenic, it causes cancer. The obvious way for drinkers to stay safe is to stop drinking. The study *Alcohol use and burden for 195 countries and territories, 1990–2016: a systematic analysis for the Global Burden of Disease Study 2016* says very clearly, "Alcohol use is a leading risk factor for global disease burden and causes substantial health loss. We found that the risk of all-cause mortality, and of cancers specifically, rises with increasing levels of consumption, and the level of consumption that minimises health loss is zero."[52] The World Health Organization states, "The harmful use of alcohol is a component cause of more than 200 disease and injury conditions in individuals, most notably alcohol dependence, liver cirrhosis, cancers and injuries."[53] But the NHS, unhelpfully says, "To keep health risks from alcohol to a low level if you drink most weeks: men and women are advised not to drink more than 14 units a week on a regular basis."[54] Surely if alcohol causes cancer the sensible advice would be to not drink it.

Harm to the liver

---

[51] *Alcohol and breast cancer risk,* Breast Cancer Now,
https://breastcancernow.org/information-support/have-i-got-breast-cancer/breast-cancer-causes/alcohol-breast-cancer-risk [17.3.21]

[52] *Alcohol use and burden for 195 countries and territories, 1990–2016: a systematic analysis for the Global Burden of Disease Study 2016,* The Lancet, https://www.thelancet.com/journals/lancet/article/PIIS0140-6736(18)31310-2 [17.3.21]

[53] *Management of substance abuse,* World Health Organization,
https://www.who.int/substance_abuse/facts/alcohol/en/ [17.3.21]

[54] *The risks of drinking too much,* NHS, https://www.nhs.uk/live-well/alcohol-support/the-risks-of-drinking-too-much [17.3.21]

The liver does much of the complicated work of removing alcohol from our system and it is a fantastic piece of equipment. This rubbery organ, weighing about 1.5kg, cleans the blood that comes from the digestive tract so it can be reused. It deals with the toxic chemicals, including alcohol, and breaks down drugs, passing the waste back into the intestines. This sophisticated organ also makes proteins for blood clotting and other functions. It converts nutrients into substances we can use, stores them and then delivers them when we need them. It also helps our blood sugar level stay constant by removing excess sugar from the blood, and it works with the kidneys to expel some waste through our urine. Every time we drink alcohol we cause the liver to work hard to get rid of the toxic chemical we introduced into our system. Regular drinking causes the liver to work extremely hard, which damages it and limits its ability to recover.[55]

As well as the risk of cancer there are a range of conditions that are the result of alcohol damage to the liver. Fatty liver disease is caused by regular drinking and a build-up of fatty cells. Hepatitis can result from binge drinking or heavy drinking and can be life threatening. Cirrhosis is a condition in which the liver cannot function due to scar tissue. The NHS says, "A person who has alcohol-related cirrhosis and does not stop drinking has a less than 50% chance of living for at least 5 more years."[56]

General harms

The list of potential harms that alcohol use can lead to includes damage to personal physical health, diseases and deaths, accidents, damage to relationships, mental health problems, damage to family networks, impacts on job security and financial difficulties. The study *Drug harms in the UK: a multicriteria decision analysis* which reviewed 20 drugs and the harms they

---

[55] *How does the liver work*, Institute for Quality and Efficiency in Health Care, https://www.ncbi.nlm.nih.gov/books/NBK279393/ [17.3.21]

[56] *Alcohol-related liver disease*, NHS, https://www.nhs.uk/conditions/alcohol-related-liver-disease-arld/ [17.3.21]

cause to the individual, as well as the harm caused to others found that alcohol was by far the most harmful drug with a harm score of 72 against 55 for heroin and 54 for crack cocaine.[57]

Unsurprisingly the alcohol industry did not appreciate this result and employed their usual tactic of blaming the individual drinkers for the damage caused by the toxic substance that they sell. The BBC article quoted Gavin Partington, of the Wine and Spirit Trade Association, who said alcohol abuse affected "a minority" who needed "education, treatment and enforcement... Clearly alcohol misuse is a problem in the country and our real fear is that, by talking in such extreme terms, Professor Nutt [one of the authors of the study] and his colleagues risk switching people off from considering the real issues and the real action that is needed to tackle alcohol misuse,"[58] he said. His use of the phrase "alcohol misuse" is biased in favour of using a moderate amount of alcohol. The real action that is needed to tackle alcohol use is to tell people they shouldn't drink it. He is wrong to say that a study that found that alcohol is harmful is "extreme."

Alcohol damages tissues in the digestive system, interfering with the natural process of digestion, preventing the body from absorbing vitamins and nutrients. Because alcohol is a poisonous harmful chemical it can cause a multitude of minor issues in our gut including gassiness, bloating and diarrhea. Long term it can lead to ulcers, hemorrhoids and internal bleeding. Alcohol also damages the digestive glands as it causes enzymes produced by the pancreas to malfunction, which can lead to pancreatitis. The pancreas also regulates the body's insulin use so damage can interfere with sugar levels in blood leading to effects and complications relating to diabetes. If our digestion doesn't work as it should we can become anemic which causes

[57] *Drug harms in the UK: a multicriteria decision analysis,* David Nutt et al. The Lancet, https://www.thelancet.com/journals/lancet/article/PIIS0140-6736(10)61462-6/ [17.3.21]

[58] *Alcohol 'more harmful than heroin' says Prof David Nutt,* BBC News, https://www.bbc.co.uk/news/uk-11660210 [17.3.21]

us to feel fatigue.

It is not surprising that the effect of a poisonous chemical on the brain can be dramatic and can lead to permanent brain damage. Wernicke-Korsakoff syndrome is a brain disorder that affects memory and is caused by drinking alcohol. Alcohol also increases the risk of dementia. The Alzheimer's Society says, "Alcohol consumption in excess has well-documented negative effects on both short- and long-term health, one of which is brain damage that can lead to Alzheimer's disease or other forms of dementia... Individuals who drank heavily or engaged in binge drinking - where a person consumes a large quantity of alcohol in a short time period - were more likely to develop Alzheimer's disease or any other form of dementia than those who engaged in moderate alcohol consumption."

Adding a toxic chemical into the blood is obviously harmful, and can lead to high blood pressure, heart problems and strokes. Our blood system is another amazing aspect of the way our bodies work, carrying oxygen to where it is needed, moving nutrients around, removing carbon dioxide and protecting us from harm. It works best as nature designed it, not infused with alcohol and we should expect the presence of a poison to have a major impact on its function.

Drinking has an impact on our reproductive system interfering with both male and female hormones, which can lead to infertility and problems in pregnancy. Women that drink while pregnant can cause long term damage to their children. Our bodies work hard to ensure we are in perfect tip top condition for the work and play that we engage in, strengthening our bones and muscles to adapt to whatever we do. Alcohol causes these subtle changes to work less effectively and drinkers may find their bones are weaker and less developed than in a healthy human. The immune system works to fight off viruses, infections and potential harms. When we drink we damage this natural protection and become more susceptible to germs and bugs. Drinkers are also more likely to develop TB and pneumonia.[59]

The World Health Organization says, "alcohol is a causal factor in more than 200 disease and injury conditions. Overall 5.1 % of the global burden of disease and injury is attributable to alcohol... Alcohol consumption causes death and disability relatively early in life. In the age group 20–39 years approximately 13.5 % of the total deaths are alcohol-attributable... There is a causal relationship between harmful use of alcohol and a range of mental and behavioural disorders, other noncommunicable conditions as well as injuries."[60] Each of us will know someone who has been harmed in some way either directly or indirectly by alcohol consumption. Our personal experience of the potential harms includes personal injuries, deaths, illnesses, cancer and accidental damage caused while drunk. We know how dangerous it is and we have all witnessed the effects, close to home, but still we drink it.

[59] Ann Pietrangelo, *The Effects of Alcohol on Your Body*, Healthline, https://www.healthline.com/health/alcohol/effects-on-body [17.3.21]

[60] *Alcohol*, World Health Organization, https://www.who.int/news-room/fact-sheets/detail/alcohol [17.3.21]

15

The addictive properties of alcohol

The World Health Organization's page about alcohol starts with this clear text: "Alcohol is a toxic and psychoactive substance with dependence producing properties,"[61] In short, alcohol is a highly addictive drug. Each alcoholic drink produces a chemical change in the drinker that the drinker feels as a mild euphoria, and as that feeling wears off the drinker will feel the need for another drink. The alcohol is an anesthetic and has the effect of reducing anxiety and numbing the senses. At the same time though the body's natural defences respond to the anesthetic by producing stress hormones including cortisol. The alcohol wears off much quicker than the cortisol, causing the drinker to feel anxious and edgy. Another drink appears to relieve the anxious and edgy feeling. This anesthetises the drinker again while causing the body to produce more cortisol. We all know the feeling of finishing a glass of wine or beer and soon after announcing it's time for another drink. It feels like a free choice but this is the effect of the alcohol wearing off. The idea to have another drink is not purely a free choice, it's the result of withdrawal.

The effect of drinking alcohol is a strange combination of downer and upper

---

[61] *Alcohol*, World Health Organisation, https://www.who.int/health-topics/alcohol [17.3.21]

as our body produces cortisol to counter the effect of the alcohol.[62] Alcohol is poisonous to humans and has a detrimental effect on our mental and physical wellbeing. As our body tries to keep us alert by producing cortisol we experience the mild euphoric buzz of the stress chemical as it raises our heart rate. This unnatural balancing act soon goes wrong because the alcohol wears off very quickly but the cortisol is present in our system for some time. Cortisol takes hours to wear off[63] but alcohol typically leaves the system at a rate of one drink per hour.[64]

The day after drinking the drinker will still have increased levels of cortisol in his or her system. This produces a feeling of anxiety and edginess the next day, and in some cases for a few days after drinking. When the anxious drinker has the first drink of the day, the alcohol will temporarily relieve the anxiety. The anesthetic effect of the alcohol calms the nerves but each drink also causes the body to produce more cortisol which continues the cycle and makes the drinker feel edgy. Each drink consumed by a drinker reinforces the idea that an alcoholic drink is relaxing or that it "takes the edge off". It is important though to understand that alcohol makes drinkers feel edgy and anxious, and then relieves the anxiety.

To make this clear, alcohol provides relief from anxiety, but causes anxiety, then provides relief from anxiety, but causes anxiety, then provides relief from anxiety.

---

[62] Ellena Badrick et al. *The Relationship between Alcohol Consumption and Cortisol Secretion in an Aging Cohort*, The Journal of Clinical Endocrinology & Metabolism, https://www.ncbi.nlm.nih.gov/pmc/articles/PMC2266962/ [17.3.21]

[63] *How long does the increased cortisol stay in your body after a stressful situation?*, Quora, https://www.quora.com/How-long-does-the-increased-cortisol-stay-in-your-body-after-a-stressful-situation [17.3.21]

[64] Dan Wagener ed. *How Long Does Alcohol Stay in Your System?*, https://americanaddictioncenters.org/alcoholism-treatment/how-long-in-system [17.3.21]

Relief is defined as "a feeling of reassurance and relaxation following release from anxiety or distress" which perfectly describes the experience that drinkers get. When a drinker feels anxiety, a drink provides "relaxation and reassurance." This appears to be a pleasurable experience but relief refers to the removal of discomfort. If we had to spend the day limping because we were walking around in shoes that were too tight, we would feel relief when we could finally take the bloody shoes off. We wouldn't wear them again because we'd recognise the cause of the discomfort. The relief that alcohol provides is less easy to identify as a source of discomfort though because of the beliefs we hold about it. We wouldn't put the too tight shoes on again just to feel relief when we take them off. But drinkers drink again and again believing that the relief that the alcohol provides is a pleasurable experience. Drinkers will know the feeling as they take the first sip of sensing a lift in their mood. But this sensation is purely in the mind. Alcohol takes more than five minutes to reach the brain when we drink but the relief appears to be immediate.

Every drinker knows the experience of going to the pub for a drink or two and waking up in the morning with the hangover from hell, thinking how did one drink turn into a skinfull? Or the experience of opening a bottle of wine to have a glass with dinner then looking at the empty bottle thinking how did I end up drinking all that? Every drinker has had to put the brakes on to stop themselves having another drink. "I can't have another, I have to work in the morning." The need for another drink is such a normal part of the drinking experience that drinkers don't question it. Imagine eating a perfect, satisfying sandwich and thinking that was a lovely, filling meal then finding a sudden desire for a sandwich, 45 minutes after you finished the last one. What stops drinkers drinking? Either they feel alarmingly drunk and recognise the danger signs and refuse more alcohol, or their responsibilities get in the way and cause them to stop.

Addictive substances are often downgraded by their users who don't like to admit to being the victim of a substance that controls them. There is a tendency to describe the regular use of an addictive drug as a habit. Here's a confusing quote from a serious study about smoking: "Smoking is a gained habit with which one starts experimenting at the age of 10, and it usually becomes part of the habit at the age of 20. It is the combination of narcotic addiction and deep-seated smoking habits."[65] Smoking though is not a habit, it is the result of the addictive properties of nicotine. Nobody is in the habit of smoking 20 cigarettes a day because a habit is a free choice, and smoking 20 cigarettes a day is the result of nicotine withdrawal, and the relief provided by each new dose of nicotine.

A habit is a routine behaviour. I eat avocado on toast at 12.00 every day and this is a habit that I have developed because I like avocado on toast and I don't eat breakfast, so I tend to be hungry at 12.00. Regular consumption of alcohol is not a habit because it is the result of the addictive properties of alcohol. Drinking a bottle of wine every evening, opening a can of lager when the drinker gets home from work, or having a glass of port after every meal is not a habit. The alcohol is addictive and the behaviour is not a free choice but the result of external factors.

Drinkers, obviously, are reluctant to accept that alcohol is addictive, and alcohol producers sell wine, beer and spirits by marketing them as sophisticated products, without mentioning how addictive they are. Oddly though, even though night after night drinkers drink more than they intended to, or got drunker than they planned to, sensed they were out of control in some way, they don't like to accept that their consumption might not have been the result of their own free will. The truth is that one drink leads to another drink which leads to another. The bottles of wine, beer and spirits that we consume are marketed to us as quality products. They don't carry warning labels like the ones on the sides of cigarette packets. You won't see a protective label

---

[65] Brankica Juranić et al. *Smoking Habit and Nicotine Effects*
https://www.intechopen.com/books/smoking-prevention-and-cessation/smoking-habit-and-nicotine-effects [17.3.21]

telling you "Warning: this wine is addictive. Consumption of one glass is likely to lead you to have another glass."

EUCAM, The European Centre for Monitoring Alcohol Marketing, exists to monitor alcohol marketing and is independent from the alcohol industry. In 2014 it produced a report entitled *The seven key messages of the alcohol industry*, which highlights the way that the alcohol industry promotes drinking. It includes this no nonsense content:

> *The industry does not draw attention to the fact that alcohol (ethanol) is a detrimental, toxic, carcinogenic and addictive substance that is foreign to the body... Chemically, alcohol is a hard drug—a substance harmful to the body, which like heroin, can cause physical and mental dependence. The reality of the negative health effects is in direct contradiction to the industry's depiction of the consumer as responsible, social, happy and celebrating life with alcohol. Alcohol is carcinogenic... No safe limit of alcohol use has been identified in relation with cancer.*[66]

Because alcohol is addictive, drinkers drink more than they should do, and drink more often than they should. Drinkers also tend to drink more in each session, becoming binge drinkers, or drinking more regularly over time. Heavy drinkers at the stage of drinking a bottle of wine every night, or binge drinking regularly know all too well that they never planned to drink that much. Nobody ever hit the legal age where they could drink and made a decision to drink a bottle of wine every night or to drink to excess and black out once a week. This increasing intake is a feature of the addictive nature of alcohol and the way that the body reacts to the consumption of alcohol.

---

[66] *The Seven Key Messages of the Alcohol Industry, Information for everyone who wants to be aware of the real intentions of the alcohol industry,* EUCAM.

The drinker's first ever alcoholic drink causes his or her body to produce a small hit of cortisol, the stress chemical that is supposed to keep us alert during times when we are under threat. As we drink more and more through the course of our lives our bodies become better at countering the threat of the alcohol and produce more cortisol, so that we feel increasingly anxious when the alcohol wears off. So a drinker that has consumed alcohol for 20 years is going to find that the substance is much more addictive than someone who is just starting to drink. How do drinkers feel the day after drinking? Slightly anxious, moderately anxious or extremely anxious, depending if their intake over time has been minimal, moderate or extreme.

Imagine going to the pub and feeling very thirsty. You stride up to the bar, "Barman, I am sooooo thirsty, I'll have a cooling pint of iced water." You take your pint of water and drink it slowly feeling the thirst quenching properties of the water. But 45 minutes after you went to the bar for your cooling pint of water, you suddenly feel the same need for the same drink, and back you go to the bar. "Barman, I will have another pint of water please." and you repeat the process. Between 6pm and midnight you end up drinking eight pints of water! This scenario does not happen, because water is not addictive and after the first pint you wouldn't be thirsty, but this is the pattern of alcohol consumption. Drinkers don't question the addictive nature of the substance that appears to be pleasurable. There is pleasure in the experience of being in the pub with your friends, or being at dinner with your partner, at parties and social events but the pleasure is not in the addictive drug that you consume. The consumption of drink after drink is caused by the withdrawal effect as the alcohol wears off. Each drink causes the drinker to need another dose of alcohol to counter the unpleasant feeling of the stress hormones.

Responsibilities

One key thing that stops drinkers drinking too much are their responsibilities. We typically see increased problematic use of alcohol when drinkers find that their responsibilities are no longer an impediment. The holiday is a good example, when there's no need to turn up to work every day and the drinker experiences true freedom for a couple of weeks. The holiday drinking often starts at the airport and continues during the holiday, starting much earlier each day than if the drinkers were in their day to day environment. It's no surprise that pensioners and the recently retired are affected by problem drinking. The pressures of daily work have gone and there is suddenly new freedom from being jobless, financially comfortable and free of children. As a result, around one fifth of all attendees at Alcoholics Anonymous are retirees.[67]

---

[67] Kerry Nenn, *Who's Going to AA? Inquiring Minds Want to Know*, American Addiction Centres, https://www.recovery.org/whos-going-to-aa-inquiring-minds-want-to-know/ [17.3.21]

16

Control

Humans are happiest when we are free to choose our own path in life. Our natural state allows us to be free to make decisions and decide our own destiny, within the confines of social and moral norms. Personal freedom is a cornerstone of much of the cultural and political thinking in the West, and our punishments tend to involve these freedoms being taken from us, if and when we break the law. Even as children our parents use the threat of being grounded, or of having the freedom to access technology or games taken from us. As adults we can be imprisoned if we break the law, resulting in our having to give up some aspect of control over our lives. Prison is the ultimate punishment, with the state in total control of the prisoner's life.

Individually, if we don't like our job, we can change it, don't like our living arrangements, we can change them, don't like our relationships, we can change them. At any time in our lives each of us are free to make choices. If an individual is unhappy then he or she has the capacity to improve their situation by making choices. We tend to be unhappy when we feel trapped, or when we feel that we are not in control. Individuals who feel trapped in a relationship may be angry or violent, and feeling trapped in a job leads to feelings of stress and anxiety.

Addictive drugs exercise a degree of control over individuals that use them.

Smoking is a great example, as smokers smoke cigarette after cigarette because they don't like the feeling of nicotine withdrawal. Each smoker is driven to smoke a cigarette between 10 and 20 times each day because of the addictive power of nicotine. They tell themselves and others that there is pleasure in smoking but deep down they know that they are a victim and would prefer to be a non-smoker. Cigarettes are poisonous to humans, they make smokers smell nasty, and they provide no benefit. Every smoker is not in control of their tobacco intake.

Because alcohol is addictive, when drinkers drink, they tend to drink more than they planned to. The addictive nature of alcohol means that after one glass of wine or beer, withdrawal causes the drinker to want to drink again, and at that moment the drinker either gives up control and accepts another drink, or they stop. Every drinker has had the experience of planning to drink one drink, and then ending up drinking more. This battle for control pitches the drinker against the addictive power of alcohol. The difficulty is that one drink causes the drinker to want to drink again at the same time that it negatively affects the drinker's judgement and self-control. This is a difficult battle to win. Every drinker has had the experience of looking back on the night before, seeing themselves as being out of control, and wondering at what point they lost control. The obvious answer is that the drinker lost control as soon as they accepted the first drink.

Alcohol is part of the fabric of our social experience and is seen as an essential part of our socialising, a key aspect of our group celebrations - think champagne and other sparkling wines at weddings, and a part of the experience of eating out - wine is marketed to us as a product that we should drink with our posh meal to show how sophisticated we are. As a drinker we are told via alcohol marketing, by our peers and by the media that we should be drinking, that the consumption of alcohol is sophisticated, traditional and classy, but time and time again we have a negative experience when we drink. It tastes nasty, it makes us feel bad and we end up drinking too much, again and again. This tension causes us to feel that we are not in control. There is pressure on each of us to drink and that pressure is another aspect where we feel as individuals we may not be fully in control. When we feel pressure to drink wine with dinner, champagne at a wedding or lager in the pub before a football match, even though we know it will be detrimental then the simple, and obvious way to exercise control is for each of us to refuse the alcohol.

I counsel drinkers who are the stage where their consumption of alcohol is a problem and I work with these individuals to try to change their beliefs about alcohol. The counselling session ends with the individual fully convinced that consuming alcohol is a negative activity, and there are no benefits to drinking. Then that individual will spend time in the same circle of friends, and the same networks, where everybody they know will try to pressure them into drinking again. Drinkers do not enjoy the total experience of drinking and yet they collectively aim to recruit more people to join them in consuming alcohol. Drinkers don't like it when someone breaks rank and refuses to drink. The reason for this is that every drinker knows they are not in control and they feel jealous of individuals that control their intake by refusing to drink.

Drinkers that moderate their intake believe that they are in control of their drinking. It's tempting to believe that the drinkers that just have one glass of wine with dinner, or one drink in the pub, are in control of their drinking. Drinking one glass of an addictive drug though means the drinker has to exercise control to not drink more. The minimal amount of alcohol they consume has a negative impact on their conversational ability, their judgement and their coordination. And there will be times when they fail to exercise control and will end up drunk. The people who look like they are in control by drinking less are not in control. They are clearly not as far down the line as the problem drinkers that have lost everything and live on the streets in the city centre but all drinkers are victims of the addictive power of alcohol.

Every drinker lost control as soon as they developed a taste for drinking alcohol. The belief that drinking is beneficial in some way, that it is essential for social interaction, that it helps with shyness, that it gives you confidence, that you need to drink it to celebrate, are all false and are beliefs peddled by drinkers. Every regular drinker has given up some element of control, and is less happy than an equivalent non-drinker.

The obvious way for drinkers to get control of their drinking is to refuse to drink alcohol. Non-drinkers do not feel pressured into drinking, do not consume a poisonous substance that affects their judgement and causes them to feel unsteady, even though the people around them tell they have to. Non-drinkers do not need to drink rotten grape juice with a nice meal, under pressure from a sommelier or some posh people who recommended a chablis over a rioja. Non-drinkers keep their focus and their conversational ability perfect at social events, and enjoy weddings without drinking a fizzy overpriced addictive drug that the people around them pressured them into drinking. "You have to have champagne to toast the bride!" Non-drinkers don't go out intending to have one glass and get home blind drunk, out of control, the result of the powerful addictive nature of alcohol.

Wine

Producers of wine and other alcohol produced from grapes stress the heritage, the exclusivity, the production methods and the craftsmanship more than any other sector. The marketing and mystique works, resulting in an army of amateur wine buffs and pseudo-experts who believe they are knowledgeable about wines and the varying tastes and subtleties of what they drink. The truth is that most of us don't have a clue what is good or bad, we couldn't tell the difference between a £10 and £100 bottle of wine, and in some cases if we are blindfolded, or if wine is cooler or warmer than usual we can't even tell a white from a red. The wine trade is a monumental con, as producers of foul tasting rotten grape juice have conned the public into paying big sums for an addictive drug. The relief of the first sip of wine feels like pleasure but as the evening wears on and drinkers get less coherent, and less good at conversation, does it matter that the wine came from a certain part of France, or that it was the result of a particularly warm year, or had a nutty nose?

Wine works well before a meal and it works during a meal, but it isn't as effective after a meal, because as drinkers' stomachs fill with food the alcohol doesn't travel to the bloodstream as easily. We all know how easily we can get pissed on an empty stomach, and obviously if our stomachs are full the alcohol we drink is less effective. Wine buffs don't like the diminishing strength of the wine they consume with meals, but luckily the wine trade has come up with a solution in fortified wine and digestifs, which are typically drunk after dinner. Wine is around 13% alcohol and is consumed during the course of a meal but once the meal is over and the drinker is full of food they need stronger drinks to deliver the same concentration of alcohol to the bloodstream. Fortified wines include port, sherry, madeira and certain dessert wines. They are artificially strengthened via the addition of more alcohol (often brandy is used, or a distilled wine) to ensure that the drinker with a full stomach gets the benefit of the alcohol. The alcohol content is much higher than wine at 20%.

Here's how The Spruce Eats website describes fortified wine:

> "A fortified wine is a delicious, viscous wine-based sipping treat. The original use of fortification was to preserve the wine, as casks of wine were prone to turn to vinegar during long sea voyages. The spirit added might also enhance the wine's natural flavors. The liquor is added to the base wine during fermentation. This fortifying of the wine brings the average alcohol content up to around 17 to 20 percent alcohol by volume."[68]

This description is typical of winespeak and I would question the fact that it is delicious and a treat. Ice cream is a treat. You probably have to sip fortified wine because it tastes nasty, being more alcoholic. The added alcohol certainly doesn't "enhance the wine's natural flavours" but it does make it more toxic. Remember that the alcohol industry constantly reinforces the idea of years

---

[68] Stacy Slinkard, *Fortified Wine Types and Uses*, The Spruce Eats, https://www.thespruceeats.com/what-is-a-fortified-wine-3510908 [17.3.21]

of tradition and craft to support the idea that alcohol is a quality product. In this case "casks of wine.. on long sea voyages" is meant to sound romantic and traditional. I would argue that drinkers don't drink port before a meal because it is too strong and gets them too pissed, but after the meal it's the perfect strength to cut through the heavy meal, and they are happy to put up with the foul taste, to ensure that the alcohol has the desired effect on them.

17

Comparing addictive drugs

There are four addictive drugs that humans consume in massive quantities: alcohol, cocaine, opiates and nicotine. Although each drug has major differences in the way they are controlled, produced and sold, they share a common feature that has led to their runaway success. Once the user of each drug has got past the initial barriers of entry, regular use settles into a pattern where the drug provides relief from withdrawal, which the user perceives as a positive feeling, followed by withdrawal, which leads to the user taking another dose. The behaviour is repetitive and the intake of the drug is determined by the speed at which the body processes the drug.

The amount of money we spend on each of these drugs is phenomenal, as is the fallout from each in terms of the number killed by these substances each year. In the US alone the public spends $253,800,000,000 ($253 billion)[69] every year on alcohol, which kills around 38,500 people[70]. The annual spend on cocaine in the US is around 10% of what is spent on alcohol at

[69] U.S. Beverage Alcohol Spending Hits $253.8 Billion in 2018, +5.1% versus 2017, BW166, https://www.bw166.com/2019/01/13/u-s-beverage-alcohol-spending-hits-253-8-billion-in-2018-5-1-versus-2017/ [17.3.21]

[70] Annual Average for United States 2011-2015 Alcohol-Attributable Deaths Due to Excessive Alcohol Use, National Center for Chronic Disease Prevention and Health Promotion, Division of Population Health, https://nccd.cdc.gov/DPH_ARDI/default/default.aspx [17.3.21]

$24,000,000,000 ($24 billion)[71], which kills 14,500 of its users[72]. Americans spend $43,000,000,000 ($43 billion) on heroin[73] and this kills 15,000 as a result[74] [75]. Tobacco use leads Americans to spend $100,300,000,000 ($100 billion) a year[76] and this results in 480,000 dead smokers every year.[77]

Nicotine

Nicotine is the drug found in tobacco and it is highly addictive. When a smoker inhales tobacco smoke the cigarette delivers a dose of nicotine, an addictive drug that provides a combination of upper and downer that the smoker experiences as a positive. The sensation of nicotine in the system is quite mild, giving smokers a slight lightheadedness and a very mild buzz. It doesn't make the smoker high or provide any benefit. As nicotine leaves the body the smoker experiences withdrawal and feels uneasy. The smoker believes that a cigarette makes them feel better so around an hour after the last cigarette is finished the smoker will light the next one, and feels relief as the negative feeling of withdrawal dissipates.

----

[71] Gregory Midgette et al. *What America's Users Spend on Illegal Drugs, 2006–2016*, Rand, https://www.rand.org/pubs/research_reports/RR3140.html [17.3.21]

[72] *Drug Overdose Deaths in the United States, 1999–2018*, NCHS Data Brief 356, Centers for Disease Control and Prevention, https://www.cdc.gov/nchs/data/databriefs/db356_tables-508.pdf [17.3.21]

[73] *What America's Users Spend on Illegal Drugs, 2006–2016*

[74] *Synthetic Opioid Overdose Data*, Centers for Disease Control and Prevention, https://www.cdc.gov/drugoverdose/data/fentanyl.html [17.3.21]

[75] *Heroin Overdose Data*, Centers for Disease Control and Prevention, https://www.cdc.gov/drugoverdose/data/heroin.html [17.3.21]

[76] *U.S. Tobacco Market Size, Share & Trends Analysis Report By Product Type (Cigarettes, Smoking Tobacco, Smokeless Tobacco, Cigars & Cigarillos), Competitive Landscape And Segment Forecasts, 2018 - 2025*, Grand View Research, https://www.grandviewresearch.com/industry-analysis/us-tobacco-market [17.3.21]

[77] *Tobacco-Related Mortality*, Centers for Disease Control and Prevention, https://www.cdc.gov/tobacco/data_statistics/fact_sheets/health_effects/tobacco_related_mortality/index.htm [17.3.21]

Cocaine

Cocaine is a highly addictive drug. It causes a high (because cocaine prevents the brain from reabsorbing its own dopamine) and as the high wears off the user will feel a sense of withdrawal which will lead them to have another line (or a lungful of smoke if the cocaine is in the form of crack). The body processes cocaine quickly so around 30 minutes after the initial dose the user feels the need to have another dose. This pattern goes on until the user exercises restraint and stops, or until the cocaine runs out. Obviously because cocaine is highly addictive, its users tend not to be very good at exercising restraint.

Opiates

Opiates are highly addictive. Opium, heroin, or prescription opiates will deliver an anesthetic effect that the user experiences as a positive feeling. As the drug wears off the user will feel a sense of withdrawal which will cause them to inject or smoke or swallow the drug again. In the case of withdrawal from opiates the user may have physical symptoms including muscle twitches, chills, and other flu-like symptoms. The time between doses varies depending on the type of opiate but as an example codeine, the common form of prescription opiate in the UK, lasts for about four hours.

Alcohol

Alcohol is highly addictive. When a drinker drinks a glass of wine, or a beer, or a shot of a spirit they feel a sense of relief that they perceive as pleasurable. The drinker's body reacts to the anesthetic effect of the alcohol by releasing stress hormones including cortisol, in an effort to keep the drinker alert. The alcohol wears off around 45 minutes after consumption but the cortisol is in the system for hours. The effect on the drinker is that as the alcohol wears off they feel edgy and anxious. This state of withdrawal causes the drinker to want to drink again and this pattern continues until the user is too drunk to drink more, or controls their intake and stops. The next day the drinker feels anxious because cortisol is still in their system and the first drink of the day appears to provide relief again.

The four drugs listed above each have unique features and are taken by very different groups of people in different circumstances but they each share the property of creating a cycle of use through providing relief, which leads to withdrawal, and in turn providing relief, then withdrawal. Essentially, addictive drugs, through regular use, work on the people that use them to make the user think there is a benefit to taking them. They trick users into believing that there is pleasure in consuming them.

Consider the way that users describe the effects of each of these drugs and compare them to what a non-user would say about them. A smoker says that smoking relieves stress and is relaxing, but if you asked a non-smoker to smoke a cigarette and report the effects he or she would tell you it made them feel dizzy and lightheaded, and that it had no effect on their stress and relaxation . A regular user of opiates will tell you it makes them feel good, and they like the feeling but a non-user would report that it made them feel tranquilised and unable to function normally. Cocaine users will tell you that coke is a social drug and that it makes them feel confident and alert but a non-user taking the drug for the first time would report that it made them feel hyper-active and jittery, and may feel overwhelmed in a social situation. Drinkers will tell you that drinking is relaxing and de-stresses them and that is essential for a social situation but non-drinkers would report that a drink made them feel unsteady, less in control, and possibly feeling sick.

We tend to think of alcohol as being different to other drugs. Commentators often talk of "drugs and alcohol" as if they are different things. Because alcohol is legal, and thanks to sophisticated marketing by the alcohol industry, its consumption is normalised. We don't tend to think of it as a substance that has parallels with illegal drugs, or to tobacco. The public perception of alcohol as a harmful addictive substance is unlikely when it is seen as a status symbol, or an essential part of a posh meal in a restaurant, or a necessary part of our celebrations.

Winners and losers

If we look at the total supply chain, production, distribution and use of each of these addictive drugs it's easy to identify who the winners and losers are. Users of addictive drugs that give up an element of control, cause themselves mental and physical harm or allow the drug to interfere with their relationships and responsibilities are victims. The corporations, drug dealers and supply chains that move drugs into the hands of the users profit from the addictive nature of the drug and are the winners.

Tobacco companies buy their crop from growers in sunny climates including India, China and Brazil. Tobacco is packaged and sold as cigarettes, rolling tobacco and powdered tobacco for chewing, and sold legally in every country worldwide. The global annual spend on tobacco is $814 billion[78] which provides an income to all the parties in the supply chain, from the shops that sell tobacco products to the manufacturers and their shareholders and employees, growers of tobacco, distributors, and the governments that receive taxation in the markets where tax is applied. These are the winners, the organisations and individuals that profit from selling tobacco. The losers are the approximately 1.1 billion smokers that consume the product. The victims of nicotine addiction spend the staggering sum of $815 billion each year poisoning themselves by consuming an addictive drug that provides no benefit. Half of all smokers die of smoking and the annual death toll is eight million as a result of smoking.[79] [80]

Cocaine is produced from coca leaf, grown in the higher regions of Peru, Bolivia and Colombia, distributed globally by criminal networks and then sold by dealers in most countries in the world who circumvent local law. There is a very small legal market for pharmaceutical cocaine which is used as

---

[78] *The global market,* BAT, https://www.bat.com/group/sites/UK___9D9KCY.nsf/vwPagesWebLive/DO9DCKFM [17.3.21]

[79] *Tobacco,* World Health Organization,
https://www.who.int/news-room/fact-sheets/detail/tobacco [17.3.21]

[80] Clive Bates and Andy Rowell, *Tobacco Explained,* Action on Smoking and health, https://www.who.int/tobacco/media/en/TobaccoExplained.pdf [17.3.21]

a topical anesthetic but this is dwarfed by the global illegal market which is estimated to be around $120 billion. This sum is shared between the growers, distributors, local dealers, and groups of individuals involved in the smuggling and movement of cocaine worldwide. These individuals are the winners and each take a share of the $120 billion[81] spent by the losers. The losers are the approximately 23 million[82] consumers of cocaine worldwide who consume the drug because it is addictive. It is difficult to find accurate numbers of global deaths from cocaine use but the figure quoted earlier in this chapter of 14,500 deaths in the US is indicative.

Opiate use globally includes a number of drugs, legal and illegal, that are produced from the opium poppy, including heroin, fentanyl, morphine, opium, and codeine. Opiates are prescribed by doctors under strict controls as pain killers and used in a medical context for managing pain. They are also produced, distributed and sold illegally outside of the legal channels by criminal networks. In some cases the legal and legitimate products produced by pharmaceutical companies are distributed via illegal channels by dealers. It is difficult to find a global figure for non-medical, illicit use of opiates but the global market for heroin is $55 billion and includes 15 million users.[83] The legal opioid market is estimated at $25 billion[84] and some of this product will be used in a non-medical setting. The winners in this market are the illegal distributors and producers of heroin and fentanyl in the markets where they are produced, the distributors of the illegal product worldwide, and local

---

[81] *Spending on Illegal Drugs*, Worldometer, https://www.worldometers.info/drugs/ [17.3.21]

[82] *Number of cocaine users worldwide from 2010 to 2018, by region*, Statista, https://www.statista.com/statistics/264738/number-of-worldwide-users-of-cocaine-by-region/ [17.3.21]

[83] *The Global Heroin Market*, World Drug Report 2010, https://www.unodc.org/documents/wdr/WDR_2010/1.2_The_global_heroin_market.pdf [17.3.21]

[84] *Opioids Market Size, Share & Trends Analysis Report By Product (IR/ Short-acting, ER/Long-acting), By Application (Pain Relief, Anesthesia), By Region, And Segment Forecasts, 2019 - 2026*, Grand View Research, https://www.grandviewresearch.com/industry-analysis/opioids-market [17.3.21]

dealers that supply the drug to users. The legal producers including Perdue Pharma, Johnson and Johnson, and others in the US and worldwide are facing lawsuits in a number of US states for their activities, and have benefitted from massive annual income as a result of use of their drugs. The losers in this transaction are the users of these highly illegal drugs who become dependent on them. 47,000 Americans overdosed and died from legal opioids in 2017[85] and the total death toll that year for all opiate users is estimated at 110,000.[86]

Alcohol producers supply an overpriced addictive, harmful legal drug, and make huge profits as a result. Alcohol production worldwide is dominated by a small number of corporations. The NGO Movendi International, which works to tackle alcohol prevention, calls these corporations "big alcohol" and puts their combined annual income at $215 billion[87]. Anheuser-Busch InBev, based in Belgium, earned $52.3 billion in 2019. These corporations are the winners in the alcohol trade, and their shareholders, suppliers and employees receive a share of their income. The smaller producers of wine, beer and spirits globally also share in the $1,470 billion ($1.47 trillion) annual spend on alcohol[88]. The losers in this transaction are the approximately 2.3 billion[89] drinkers who consume an addictive drug that harms and kills 3.3 million of them every year.

Each of these four drugs is addictive and causes harm to the people that

---

[85] *Opioid epidemic in the United States,* Wikipedia, https://en.wikipedia.org/wiki/Opioid_epidemic_in_the_United_States [17.3.21]

[86] Hannah Ritchie and Max Roser, *Opioids, cocaine, cannabis and illicit drugs,* https://ourworldindata.org/illicit-drug-use [17.3.21]

[87] *Big Alcohol Exposed,* Movendi, https://movendi.ngo/the-issues/the-problem/exposing-big-alcohol/ [17.3.21]

[88] *Size of the alcoholic beverage market worldwide from 2018 to 2024,* Statista, https://www.statista.com/statistics/696641/market-value-alcoholic-beverages-worldwide/ [17.3.21]

[89] *Global status report on alcohol and health 2018,* World Health Organisation, https://www.who.int/publications/i/item/9789241565639 [17.3.21]

use them but the market for each is also massive and the profits that result from the production, distribution and sale of each ensures that the status quo remains. The alcohol industry spends vast amounts of money on government lobbying, marketing and PR, while it also funds not-for-profit organisations that promote safe, responsible drinking. It promotes its products as sophisticated and refined, and stresses the heritage and the craftsmanship in the production of spirits such as whiskies, and wines. The alcohol industry wants to ensure that the addictive poison that it sells to its victims is legal in as many countries as possible, and subject to as little legislation as possible. Its ultimate aim is maximising profit.

Any drinker that is willing to spend large amounts of money on a bottle of wine or spirit is a victim of the alcohol industry, and has bought into the beliefs that all drinkers share - that the substance in the bottle has some quality that is worth paying for. A bottle of grape juice costs less than a pound in my local supermarket, which indicates to me that a company can pick grapes, crush grapes and bottle the juice in a good quality glass bottle and ship it to supermarkets around the UK for very little money. The same grape juice that has rotted, in a similar bottle, produced from similar grapes and shipped to the same supermarkets as wine costs a lot more, and with some fizz and a bit of foil added to the top even more as champagne. Drinkers drink alcohol because it is addictive, and they pay huge amounts for it because the alcohol industry convinced them it was sophisticated and classy. The more they drink of it, the more it harms them. This has to be the greatest con trick of all time.

18

Stress hormones

Humans are governed to some degree by chemical changes that are the result of our subconscious reacting to the world around us. Although we believe we are free thinkers and our behaviour is driven by personal choice, our reactions and reflexes exert control. Our natural system produces hormones to reward us for good behaviour, or to warn us when we are in danger. We receive serotonin and dopamine as rewards for socialising, when we fancy someone, when we have sex, when we exercise, when we discover things and when we eat nice food[90]. Nature is incentivising good human interaction, furthering the species by encouraging us to engage in behaviours that will lead to more babies being born, and rewarding us for sticking together with our peers and looking after ourselves. When we sense danger, or if we are caught up in a scary situation, or we are in conflict situations, we experience the opposite, as our system uses stress hormones to make sure that we are aware that we are in danger, to ensure we are ready for a fight or that we are ready to flee.

Our amazing brain and our system of controls and reflexes works to keep us safe by using stress hormones, produced and controlled by various parts of the

---

[90] *How Brain Chemicals Influence Mood and Health,* University of Pittsburgh Medical Center, https://share.upmc.com/2016/09/about-brain-chemicals/ [17.3.21]

brain, known as the stress response[91]. The complexity and sophistication of this system buried deep in the brain is phenomenal, signaling various levels of stress or danger to us using subtle adjustments in the release of a combination of chemicals. In simple terms, this system works via the combination of two main stress hormones, adrenaline and cortisol.

Adrenaline is the hormone that is immediate and causes us to react quickly to a scary situation. Imagine being caught in a shoot-out, or witnessing a major car crash right where you are standing. Our system uses a surge of adrenaline to make us super alert and ready to run, or take action - the fight or flight response. When we sense sudden shock we say, "I felt my heart jump!" We experience adrenaline as an immediate change that puts us on edge, but it also subsides quickly leaving us calm again. Minor things such as bad news, news of a death or crashing your bike are likely to trigger a minor surge of adrenaline. Adrenaline is the stress hormone that we associate with panic.

In conjunction with adrenaline, our brain also controls the release of cortisol, the slow release stress hormone that works to make sure we know when we are stressed. Cortisol is likely to be released when we are under pressure at work, in a challenging relationship, or when we are in a difficult situation over an extended period of time. The cortisol is released to indicate to us that we are in a non-optimal situation, but unlike adrenaline, it stays in our system for a long time, and we are likely to feel edgy and anxious for a few hours following the release of cortisol. Cortisol is always present in our system but increased stress causes increased levels that lead to anxiety, a raised heart rate, loss of appetite, and we may feel shaky or agitated. In the modern world we typically experience a busy life with competing priorities, high pressure at work, poor job security, expensive housing, and the juggling of friendships, deadlines, relationships, and a constant feed of information from our smartphones and

---

[91] *Understanding the stress response,* Harvard Health Publishing, https://www.health.harvard.edu/staying-healthy/understanding-the-stress-response [17.3.21]

screens. It's no wonder that people describe feeling stressed all the time.

The stress hormones that we experience are supposed to be temporary because ideally, we are relaxed and calm throughout our lives. When difficult situations or threats arise our subconscious brain uses stress hormones to get us through the risky period, but as the threat subsides our chemical balance is restored and we return to our calm state. Being stressed for long periods of time is bad for us and there are a number of ways that long term stress can damage our health.

Alcohol is a poisonous anesthetic and has the potential to harm us. When we drink it it causes our system of controls and reflexes to react by producing the stress hormone cortisol to keep us alert. Cortisol stays in our system for hours, and each drink we consume causes more to be released. Even though our conscious brain is convinced that we should drink alcohol, our subconscious knows full well that alcohol is dangerous and deals with the threat by releasing hormones to keep us safe. Drinkers feel anxious the day after drinking because of the increased levels of cortisol that are the result of the brain dealing with the threat of the alcohol. If we drink regularly the cortisol accumulates in our system and if we refrain from drinking the cortisol subsides. Because cortisol takes hours to return to normal levels drinkers that drink everyday will have permanently raised cortisol levels.

Drinkers produce more cortisol over time. The first alcoholic drink causes the body to produce a small amount of cortisol but as the drinker drinks again and again, the brain learns to produce more and more cortisol each time. In this way someone who has consumed 100,000 units of alcohol to date will produce more cortisol when they drink, than someone who has consumed 10,000 units. Alcohol is addictive because of the cortisol but it becomes more addictive to the drinker who has consumed more over time. A drinker in his or her mid 20s may have a higher production of cortisol as a result of their drinking than someone in their mid-60s, if the younger person has consumed a lot of alcohol during their drinking years.

There is a lot written about high levels of stress and anxiety in society and there are a myriad of causes that exacerbate mental wellbeing across the population including physical health, the quality of our relationships, availability of employment, poverty and equality. Because alcohol causes anxiety societies that have high levels of alcohol consumption will tend to have higher levels of anxiety. In the Telegraph article entitled *Boozy Britons are drinking 108 bottles of wine a year - far more than the rest of the western world*[92], the journalist points out that our alcohol consumption has increased versus a number of other comparable countries. It's no surprise that at the same time our anxiety levels and use of antidepressants have risen. The Guardian's 2017 story says it well: *NHS prescribed record number of antidepressants last year,*[93] pointing out that a record number of nearly 65 million prescriptions were handed out in one year. Anxiety in society is the result of a number of factors and alcohol isn't the only issue but it seems to be the least well understood contributor to the nation's rising levels.

The relationship between cortisol and alcohol is the key to understanding the way that alcohol works as an addictive drug, and the impact it has on regular drinkers, but it does not seem to be on the radar of the health professionals that give us advice about alcohol and what it does to us. David Nutt's books, *Drugs WIthout the Hot Air*, makes no mention of cortisol and his more recent *Drink?*, mentions the fact that cortisol seems to be a feature of withdrawal from alcohol but with no further details.

Regular drinking raises cortisol levels but these return to normal if the drinker leaves sufficient time between drinking sessions. The exact time varies. I have a friend who says she feels on edge for weeks after drinking but this is

---

[92] Laura Donnelly, *Boozy Britons are drinking 108 bottles of wine a year - far more than the rest of the western world*, The Telegraph, https://www.telegraph.co.uk/news/2019/11/07/boozy-britons-drinking-108-bottles-wine-year-far-rest-western/ [17.3.21]

[93] Denis Campbell, *NHS prescribed record number of antidepressants last year*, The Guardian, https://www.theguardian.com/society/2017/jun/29/nhs-prescribed-record-number-of-antidepressants-last-year [17.3.21]

unusual. For most people five days without a drink should be sufficient to get stress levels back to normal. If drinkers do drink daily, or regularly enough that cortisol levels are above normal they should be aware of the potential effects of being stressed for long periods of time.

Having raised levels of stress hormones in our system causes loss of appetite and this is why heavy or regular drinkers tend to be slim - they don't feel hungry. Being stressed for extended periods interferes with fertility so if you are drinking too much and struggling to get pregnant the doctor will advise you to stop drinking so that your natural reproductive system can work as it should (alcohol is obviously a very dangerous thing to consume when pregnant anyway). Being stressed also interferes with your sleep and makes it difficult to get a proper night's sleep (on top of the damage to your sleep that alcohol does). Extended periods of stress can also lead to depression, and physical problems including heart disease.[94]

Heavy drinkers that drink every day are maintaining a delicate balancing act, drinking wine, beer and spirits to calm the nerves, but finding their cortisol levels spiralling higher and higher. The alcohol has historically caused temporary relief as the anesthetic briefly makes the drinker feel calmer but as the drinker drinks more and more they experience constant anxiety and fear because the cortisol is flooding the system. Every day, heavy drinkers drink to relieve the anxiety but experience more anxiety as a result. These high levels of cortisol in the system have the potential to overwhelm the heavy drinker who experiences massive anxiety and edginess. This drives the drinker to drink a lot. I have met several heavy drinkers who say they need a drink in the morning, or at lunchtime, to calm themselves just so they can function normally at work.

If a heavy drinker who balances the stress with a regular intake of alcohol

---

94 *Chronic stress puts your health at risk*, Mayo Clinic, https://www.mayoclinic.org/healthy-lifestyle/stress-management/in-depth/stress/art-20046037 [17.3.21]

stops drinking they are going to feel the effects of the stress. They will feel shaky, panicky and anxious because of the cortisol, but the cortisol will leave the system over time and each day the drinker who refuses a drink will find themselves becoming calmer. Five days after a drink stress levels should be back to normal.

The scenario of heavy drinkers being flooded with stress hormones seems to not be well understood by the medical profession. Advice from medical professionals talks of DTs, delirium tremens, a mysterious case of the shakes, or possibly seizures, as a result of what is sometimes called alcohol withdrawal syndrome. A number of websites that detail the likely symptoms of giving up drinking include an elevated heart rate, anxiety, sweating, the shakes, etc. These are typical of highly stressed individuals. The US National Library of Medicine's Medline Plus website includes the following advice, which doesn't mention stress: "Delirium tremens can occur when you stop drinking alcohol after a period of heavy drinking, especially if you do not eat enough food... [it] may also be caused by head injury, infection, or illness in people with a history of heavy alcohol use. It occurs most often in people who have a history of alcohol withdrawal. It is especially common in those who drink 4 to 5 pints (1.8 to 2.4 liters) of wine, 7 to 8 pints (3.3 to 3.8 liters) of beer, or 1 pint (1/2 liter) of "hard" alcohol every day for several months. Delirium tremens also commonly affects people who have used alcohol for more than 10 years."[95]

There are examples of advice suggesting that heavy drinkers should not stop drinking suddenly and are encouraged to taper their intake. No surprise that this is often included in the advice of companies that offer rehab and care to heavy drinkers, and that charge expensive fees. Castle Craig's website says, "Quitting alcohol "cold turkey" — or by abruptly cutting off your supply — can be dangerous and, if not managed properly, will fail. Alcoholics who quit cold turkey without the care and supervision of trained medical staff are at risk for not only relapse but also serious medical conditions." but then

---

[95] *Delirium tremens*, Medline Plus, https://medlineplus.gov/ency/article/000766.htm [17.3.21]

mysteriously argues, "Your body has come to depend on sugar and grains from alcohol, so when you stop drinking cold turkey, your body craves those sugar and grains."[96]

Some drinkers are prescribed sedatives to deal with the effects of high levels of stress that are the result of stopping drinking. It would probably be helpful for a heavy drinker to understand exactly what is causing the anxiety and fear when they decide to stop drinking - it is stress, the feeling of having raised levels of cortisol in the system.

To sum up all this in basic terms, because alcohol is a poisonous anesthetic our body reacts by doing what it does best, trying to keep us safe. The threat of alcohol causes the production of the stress chemical cortisol. The cortisol in our system makes us anxious when the alcohol wears off, and this makes alcohol addictive because it causes us to want to drink again. Alcohol appears to make us relaxed and calm but this is because it provides relief, briefly, for drinkers that have increased levels of cortisol. But the cortisol is the result of drinking alcohol. This means that alcohol causes us to be anxious and fools us into thinking it relieves that anxiety. As we drink more over time we produce more cortisol, which means that alcohol becomes more addictive. Heavy drinkers balance high levels of cortisol with the alcohol they drink. When the alcohol is taken away they feel highly stressed and have physical symptoms including sweating and the shakes.

If you want to be stressed and anxious, have some drinks and once the alcohol has worn off you should feel the effect of raised levels of your natural stress hormones. More regular drinks will mean more stress and anxiety. The more you drink, the more stressed and anxious you will feel. If you like feeling calm and relaxed, stop drinking and let the stress hormones naturally deplete in

---

[96] Wagdy Fahmi, *Going Cold Turkey: The Wrong Way to Quit Alcohol*, Castle Craig, https://castlecraig.co.uk/blog/2020/01/15/going-cold-turkey-the-wrong-way-to-quit-alcohol [17.3.21]

your system. Five days should be enough to get your natural balance restored.

19

The drinking journey

Each individual's alcohol consumption over time can be compared to a one way train journey with a start point and end point. Each drinker starts the journey with their first drinking experience, encouraged by other drinkers who recruited him or her. As the drinker continues to drink, over time their intake will increase and the frequency of drinking will increase. The journey takes in a number of stops as the drinker progresses from the first drinking experience to occasional social drinking, regular social drinking, binge drinking, drinking in isolation, heavy daily drinking, drinking that causes the drinker to give up their responsibilities, etc. The final stop on the drinking journey is death (more than 3 million died from their alcohol intake in 2016[97]), which thankfully most drinkers do not get close to reaching. Drinkers progress along the line if they drink, and the more they drink the quicker they travel. I know of individuals that have died in their 20s and 30s having started drinking in their teens. Drinkers that drink less progress more slowly, and we probably all know people in their 60s and 70s who barely drink and are still in the early stages of their drinking journey.

---

[97] *Harmful use of alcohol kills more than 3 million people each year, most of them men,* World Health Organization, https://www.who.int/news/item/21-09-2018-harmful-use-of-alcohol-kills-more-than-3-million-people-each-year—most-of-them-men [17.3.21]

The key feature of the journey, that only goes one way, is that any drinker can stop drinking and get off the metaphorical train at any time. A non-drinker does not progress any further along the line but as soon as the non-drinker starts drinking again they will restart the journey at the same point they stopped at when they gave up drinking. A drinker that binges every weekend, and that stops drinking for some time, will find when they start again they quickly fall into the same pattern of binge drinking every weekend. Drinkers cannot return to the places they have left. No drinker who is a heavy daily drinker can return to the days when they had an occasional drink with friends and left it at that. We cannot become the drinker we used to be. We either drink, and travel along the line as a result, or we stop drinking and get off the train.

The four common addictive drugs are nicotine, opiates, cocaine and alcohol. Each drug has similarities in the way they cause their users to want to take the drug again when they are consuming it, but there are big differences in the effect of their users' intake over extended time periods. Alcohol has a feature that causes drinkers to progressively drink more over time. This means that as drinkers consume alcohol during their life they tend to drink more at each session, and more often, and this is because of the way that our bodies react by producing cortisol, our natural stress hormone.

Comparing cigarette smoking to alcohol consumption is a good way to illustrate the difference in the way nicotine and alcohol work. A smoker that starts smoking, at whatever age, is likely to smoke at the rate at which his or her body processes nicotine. So if a smoker has a normal body that is good at removing nicotine quickly the smoker may feel the need for the next cigarette 45 minutes after the last cigarette they smoked. This causes the smoker to light a new cigarette every 45 minutes between waking and going to bed, leading to around 20 cigarettes being smoked every day. If the smoker's system takes longer to process the nicotine, for instance taking 90 minutes between each cigarette then they are likely to smoke 10 cigarettes every day (based on these primitive calculations, it's no surprise that cigarettes come in boxes of 10 or 20). This figure doesn't change over time. A cigarette smoker that smokes 20 a day for their first year of smoking will almost certainly smoke 20 a day in their 20th year of smoking.

If you know a smoker, or have been a smoker, then you will be able to recognise this behaviour. Smoking becomes a subconscious action as it is performed so often. In the UK a packet of 20 cigarettes costs more than a decent paperback book, and it sustains the smoker for one day, causing the smoker to be less happy, to be less healthy, and to stink of cigarette smoke. All this to stave off the withdrawal from nicotine. Smokers may smoke more when they drink, or less when they are in an environment where they are banned from smoking, but without these restrictions or boosts, day to day use doesn't change, and the smoker typically smokes a consistent number every day for years before either giving up, or dying.

Alcohol has a feature that causes its users to consume more over time, and this makes the pattern of alcohol consumption very different to smoking. When we drink alcohol the anesthetic effect of the alcohol causes the body to produce the stress hormone cortisol to counter the threat of the alcohol. Each drink we drink causes our body to produce more cortisol, which makes us feel more anxious each time. We feel this the next day in our anxiety levels as the cortisol stays in our system. All drinkers' early drinking caused minimal feelings of anxiety and edginess the next day. Novice drinkers have low cortisol production as a result of drinking. The brain's subconscious system hasn't had to deal with an anesthetic poison being administered before and it is just learning what to do. As drinkers drink more and progress on the drinking journey the brain becomes more efficient and becomes better at giving us a protective dose of the stress hormone cortisol to keep us alert whenever we drink. This has the result that the more we drink, the more anxious we feel.

Heavy drinkers in the later stages of the drinking journey will find that their brain produces large quantities of cortisol and will feel anxious and on edge all day. They will spend their day looking forward to the first drink to calm the nerves, to take the edge off. The alcohol only temporarily works and the anxiety returns, causing the drinker to drink again, and again and again. The night's heavy intake causes the drinker to have another day of anxiety, and the pattern continues.

A client I counselled described his day to me, which illustrates what late stage drinking looks like: He told me he had to drink a couple of gin and tonics to calm the nerves in the morning before work, then at lunchtime he would drink wine to get him through the afternoon. Drinks in the pub after work would sustain him until he got home when he would drink another bottle of wine or two before bed. He told me if he didn't drink he felt highly stressed. Now he doesn't drink he recognises that as a drinker he believed that alcohol relieved anxiety. Now he can see that it caused anxiety.

No drinker starts their journey by drinking all day every day. We all start with an intake that seems managed and appears to be a free choice. We embark on the journey convinced that the substance in the glass is benign and part of our socialising and that it is pleasurable, even though it has such a negative effect on us when we drink it. Once we have learned to tolerate the effects, got past the stage where we vomit, and convinced ourselves that we are in control of our drinking, we are likely to move on, and as we progress we never stop to question why we are drinking or notice our intake increasing. Drinkers that open a bottle of wine every night after work, and end up consuming the whole bottle never consider that something other than their own free will may be acting on them and causing them to drink more than they used to.

At the point when a drinker decides to stop drinking, they travel no further along the drinking journey. Their natural defences though have been conditioned over time to produce massively elevated levels of stress hormones when they consume alcohol. The system has been improved and strengthened by the alcohol they have drunk to date. The natural, and highly sophisticated reflex that senses threats to the individual is now very good at reacting to alcohol and is ready for the next moment when it has to work hard to keep the drinker safe. Weeks, months or years later when the drinker picks up a drink thinking that they will control their intake like they first did when they used to enjoy the pub, the brain will flood the system with cortisol, and the drinker will immediately feel high levels of anxiety. The alcohol is now much more addictive and the drinker will experience alcohol not as they did in the early days of their drinking journey, but exactly at the same point that they stopped drinking.

20

Moderation

There is a common phrase in use that refers to acceptable levels of drug and alcohol use: everything in moderation. Attributed to Oscar Wilde, and originating from the bible, it implies that small amounts of something are OK and is often used in dieting circles. I'm partial to a biscuit but I know that to eat biscuits all day would be a problem. Eating biscuits is pleasurable. Users of drugs will argue that taking a small dose of an addictive drug is also pleasurable. The small dose that seems pleasurable to a drug user would seem unpleasant to a non-user though. A cigarette is not pleasurable to a non-smoker, an alcoholic drink is unpleasant if you force it on a non-drinker, opiates cause non-users to feel like they have been anesthetised and cocaine makes non-users feel shaky and hyperactive. A biscuit is pleasurable in small doses. Addictive drugs don't provide genuine pleasure. Everything in moderation, the idea that a small amount of a substance is OK, is not appropriate when applied to addictive drugs. A small amount of an addictive drug tends to lead to more of the addictive drug, or more regular use of the addictive drug, or more of the addictive drug being taken each time. Because of this advice to users that moderation is OK is dangerous and misguided.

If a smoker wrote a report on smoking they would say that smoking is relaxing and pleasurable. If heroin users wrote a report about heroin they would say that it is relaxing and pleasurable but don't use too much of it. Cocaine users would say that the drug is great in social situations but keep it under control. Each group of users would provide a biased report in favour of the drug being used in moderation. Drinkers have done the same. We are informed by guidance written by drinkers that downgrades alcohol from a dangerous, toxic, harmful, addictive drug to something that is fine in moderation. Use is fine to them but "misuse" is a problem. Regular alcohol use is fine but "alcohol use disorder" is a problem. The drinkers that have written the guidance have created a dangerous, and false, categorisation of drinkers into two groups, those who drink safely, and those who have lost control. This myth is repeated again and again in different ways but is a key aspect of the way we think about drinking. It is dangerous because it tells us all that moderate drinking is safe, and because every drinker considers that they are in the safe zone.

Former drug users, individuals that have abstained following a period of problem use, would produce a very different report about the drug, when compared to active users. Smokers that have given up will tell you to never start, that they hated smoking, that it made them smell disgusting, that it was a waste of money. Ex-drinkers, whether heavy drinkers or moderate drinkers, will tell you that since giving up they feel better. They will warn you that alcohol is addictive, that drinkers tend to be out of control, that there are no benefits to drinking. Ex-heroin users will certainly warn others off opiates, point out that heroin use interferes with daily responsibilities, and explain that the withdrawal is a nightmare. Ex-cocaine users will tell you very clearly how powerful the addictive properties of the drug are, and how it can quickly become a dangerous and controlling aspect of the users' life.

The simple solution to the problem of addictive drugs is simply not to take them. Moderation is bad advice and misses the obvious. To ensure that the use of a small amount of an addictive drug does not escalate into a larger amount, the user should not take the small amount. Every drinker started drinking with a small amount of alcohol in their first drinking session. Every drinker started with alcohol in moderation, and every drinker looking at their current level of consumption is aware that what started as moderation has increased over time. Moderation does not work.

21

Cutting down and time off

The majority of clients that I counsel, and who are at the later stages of the drinking journey, always have the same desire before the counselling session starts: "I would really like to just cut down, and be like the social drinker I once was." My response is to set them a challenge: "Buy a bottle of wine, take it home on a quiet evening when you are alone, and just drink one glass of wine, then cork the bottle and put it back in the fridge." Or "Buy yourself a box of 12 bottles of beer and on a quiet evening when you are alone, just have one bottle and leave the 11 other bottles in the fridge." At this point the client laughs and says this isn't possible. Drinkers at the later stages of the drinking journey find alcohol extremely addictive and once they start drinking they find it impossible to stop. The need to drink is much more powerful to them than it was when they first started drinking. The beer or wine is the same strength, but their own response to the alcohol has changed over time. They are better at producing cortisol and as a result, they are compelled to drink again and again. When this is pointed out they generally recognise they have two options available to them, to stop drinking, or continue to drink and be a victim of the powerful addictive properties of alcohol.

Almost every agency, charity, medical body and scientist that is involved in issuing guidance in the UK repeatedly trots out the same nonsensical advice about alcohol, that drinkers should try to cut down. This advice is laughable because alcohol is addictive, and the advice becomes even more laughable for drinkers that are further along the drinking journey. The heavy daily drinker cannot have a day off drinking because their anxiety levels would be through the roof. They find they have to maintain their intake just to be calm enough to get through the day. A binge drinker that drinks to excess every Friday night does have a whole week off between binges, but this isn't a useful tactic for controlling their intake because as soon as they start drinking on a Friday night the addictive power of alcohol will cause them to drink and drink and drink, to the point where they may be harmed by the alcohol, or suffer personal injuries as a result of their drunkenness.

Cutting down is a poor attempt to exercise control over an addictive drug. Imagine advising smokers to cut down, or to have a day off smoking. As soon as they light up again they start the cycle of relief and withdrawal. The only advice to smokers is to stop smoking. Try convincing a heroin user to just have a few days off, or to cut down. Heroin is highly addictive and because users build up tolerance they tend to also use more of the drug over time, and each time they use. Try using less is not good advice for heroin users. Stop taking the drug, and allow the body and mind to revert to its natural healthy state is the only advice worth giving. Suggesting to a cocaine user that regularly consumes the drug that they have a few days off is pointless. Cocaine users often have days off between using the drug but using a highly addictive drug means that when they take it they tend to consume line after line until the drug is gone. The advice to cut down is extremely unhelpful for drinkers and should be replaced with a simple message - stop drinking.

Time off

There are a number of well known branded breaks from alcohol. The obvious one is Dry January (Alcohol Change UK holds the trademark), a naturally sensible way to have a clean month after the alcohol-soaked Christmas and New Year period. According to The Week, four million people signed up to have a month off alcohol in 2020.[98] More recently One Year No Beer has established itself as a brand, promising, "Change Your Relationship With Alcohol And Watch Your Whole World Change." (this is another example of a failure to tell people not to drink. Why not "stop drinking and watch your whole world change"?) The website, an excellent exercise in branding and design sets out its stall: every drinker would feel better if they stopped drinking, and the website highlights the major improvement areas: improved sleep, feeling better, more productive, reduced anxiety and losing weight[99]. Giving up drinking for a day, a month, a week, a year, or even 20 years, is fantastic. Every drinker that stops drinking will notice an improvement. Ideally the drinker gives up for some time, figures out that they are happier, healthier, wealthier and more productive without alcohol in their lives, and then decides to not pick up a drink again. The challenge of course is the army of drinkers that pressure all of us into drinking, and that will apply peer pressure on every non-drinker, to try to get them to go back to drinking.

Every drinker will also discover that they are the same drinker that they were before they stopped, if and when they start again. If a drinker that consumes a bottle of wine every night, night after night, takes a year off, and then decides to start drinking again, they will quickly find that they settle into the same rhythm. The rate of drinking is determined by the alcohol, not by the drinker. The drinker cannot go back to become the happy go lucky consumer of alcohol that likes an occasional drink in their early days of drinking.

Each of us learnt to drink because the people around us, who were already drinkers, convinced us that we couldn't enjoy a social event without a drink in our hands. Dry January, One Year No Beer, and other similar abstinence programmes tell us the truth - that the substance we have finally stopped

---

[98] *Is Dry January really worth it?*, The Week, https://www.theweek.co.uk/62059/dry-january-what-is-it-and-is-it-actually-worth-it [17.3.21]

[99] *One Year No Beer*, https://www.oneyearnobeer.com/ [17.3.21]

consuming only did us harm. The most important thing for drinkers to learn during the period of abstinence is to not start drinking again. Dry January is short. One Year is longer. A life without alcohol is ideal.

22

Bias

The public puts a great deal of trust in the practitioners and medical experts that produce guidance to keep us safe from harm. We look to the Government to give us guidance via its own institutions such as Public Health England and the Department of Health and Social Care (DHSC), which in turn has responsibility for the National Health Service (NHS). The Government set up NICE, the National Institute for Health and Care Excellence in 1999, to advise on drugs and treatments in the NHS. It "provides national guidance and advice to improve health and social care."[100] NICE is an executive non-departmental public body, sponsored by the DHSC. Collectively these departments and organisations produce the guidance and advice that is issued to the public to keep us healthy and safe from harm. Their research and findings are based on evidence and as a result they carry a great deal of public trust. We look to the Government as a trusted advisor and we believe that the decisions they make about our collective health and wellbeing are sound.

The Government departments set policies and issue guidance on alcohol consumption as part of their remit and this guidance tends to be fed to the media when there is a press release or when something newsworthy is issued. The newspapers and websites that we rely on for daily news filter

---

[100] *About Us,* NICE, https://www.nice.org.uk/about [17.3.21]

the information and feed us the newsworthy content, which we collectively absorb. As a result, these agencies' findings become part of the lingua franca and are embedded in the way we understand and think about alcohol. We trust the established news media, and by and large we trust the government, so it makes perfect sense that we believe what we hear and we accept what we are told.

As well as the powerful combination of the government agencies and the news media there are a number of prominent charities that exist to counter the negative impact of alcohol consumption. They are backed up by a huge number of local or specialist charities which contribute to our collective understanding of alcohol and the harm it can cause. From the largest few down to the thousands of smaller ones, each charity issues guidance and advice to inform the public about their consumption. The big charities that contribute to our understanding are Drinkaware, Alcohol Change UK and Alcoholics Anonymous.

There are a number of other organisations whose guidance contributes to the public understanding of alcohol including the Alcohol Health Alliance, a "coalition of more than 50 organisations working together to reduce the harm caused by alcohol,"[101] The Portman Group, "the social responsibility body and regulator for alcohol labelling, packaging and promotion in the UK."[102] The Institute of Alcohol Studies, "an independent institute bringing together evidence, policy and practice from home and abroad to promote an informed debate on alcohol's impact on society."[103]

There are also a number of educational and research organisations including universities that contribute to our knowledge of alcohol and these include the Alcohol Research Group, part of Kings College London, University College

---

[101] *Who We Are*, Alcohol Health Alliance, https://ahauk.org/ [17.3.21]

[102] *About the Portman Group*, The Portman Group, https://www.portmangroup.org.uk/ [17.3.21]

[103] *Institute of Alcohol Studies*, http://www.ias.org.uk/ [17.3.21]

London's Tobacco & Alcohol Research Group, Sheffield Alcohol Research Group, part of the University of Sheffield and the The Drug and Alcohol Research Centre, part of Middlesex University London, as well as many more. Individuals back up this body of work in the books that are written about alcohol and the impact that it can have on us.

We are not short of advice about alcohol. The plethora of organisations listed in the paragraphs above all have an interest in issuing advice because they all share a common goal, to reduce the harmful effects of alcohol. Government money, charitable income, research grants and university fees all feed this collective, and their advice filters down into the public's understanding about alcohol. Although some research is independent, there has been an increase in research funded by alcohol companies. A recent study by the University of York found a 56% increase in research funded by alcohol companies and pointed out that 13,500 studies were found to be funded by the alcohol industry. This is likely to result in bias in the research and is a clear conflict of interest[104]. We exist in a time when there is more available advice about alcohol issued by a sector that is larger than it has ever been in the past. More agencies, more money, more charitable income, more experts, more advice and more guidance should be a good thing. The public should be safer as a result of all this money, time and effort. We should be drinking less, and we should be suffering less harm as the result of our drinking but in fact the opposite is true.

Drinking levels are at their highest ever, alcohol consumption has increased and alcohol harm is a bigger problem now than in the past. Here's an illustration from the NICE guidance *Alcohol dependence and harmful alcohol use*:

---

[104] *Increase in alcohol-industry funded research is a cause for concern, study suggests,* University of York, https://www.york.ac.uk/news-and-events/news/2020/research/alcohol-research-funding/ [17.3.21]

"The physical harm related to alcohol has been increasing in the UK in the past three decades. Deaths from alcoholic liver disease have doubled since 1980 (Leon & McCambridge, 2006) compared with a decrease in many other European countries. Alcohol related hospital admissions increased by 85% between 2002/03 and 2008/09, accounting for 945,000 admissions with a primary or secondary diagnosis wholly or partly related to alcohol in 2006/07 and comprising 7% of all hospital admissions (North West Public Health Observatory, 2010)."[105]

The guidance doesn't seem to be reducing our consumption, even though the time effort and resources within the collective organisations that are supposed to prevent us being harmed by alcohol has increased. In fact the public is drinking more, and being harmed more. This is a curious situation but there is an obvious reason for this and that is that the guidance is biased and tends to promote alcohol consumption. This bias exists because the experts that write the guidance are drinkers and because of the influence of the alcohol industry. Guidance written by drinkers causes people that shouldn't drink alcohol to continue to drink alcohol because the guidance says it is OK to drink in moderation.

A review of the output of the agencies listed above including charities, government agencies, research bodies and independent bodies reveals a simple problem, and that is that none of them advises the public not to drink alcohol. The result is that the public, who already have alcohol promoted to them by the massively powerful alcohol industry, turn to the experts and institutions that they trust and are told that it's perfectly fine to drink.

There is a rare and unusual recent piece of work that does say we shouldn't drink. Just one. The study, *Alcohol use and burden for 195 countries and*

---

[105] *Alcohol Use Disorders*, NICE, https://www.nice.org.uk/guidance/cg115/evidence/full-guideline-136423405 [17.3.21]

territories, 1990–2016: a systematic analysis for the Global Burden of Disease Study 2016, published in the Lancet in 2018 included this summary: "Alcohol use is a leading risk factor for global disease burden and causes substantial health loss. We found that the risk of all-cause mortality, and of cancers specifically, rises with increasing levels of consumption, and the level of consumption that minimises health loss is zero."[106] This makes it clear that alcohol is dangerous in any quantity. The easy way to avoid being harmed by alcohol is to not drink alcohol. EUCAM's report *The seven key messages of the alcohol industry*, calls alcohol "a detrimental, toxic, carcinogenic and addictive substance that is foreign to the body... Alcohol is carcinogenic... No safe limit of alcohol use has been identified in relation with cancer."[107] The report is not specifically about alcohol consumption, it is about the way that the alcohol industry markets their product.

Professor David Nutt, writing in *Drugs Without the Hot Air* gives us a typical example of the bias that is present in guidance produced by drinkers. In his chapter about alcohol and its harms he asks the important question: "how can we reduce the harm done by alcohol?"[108] The obvious answer would be to tell people not to drink it. Like every addictive, dangerous drug, the best way to avoid being harmed by alcohol is to not consume alcohol. Instead, David's options are to: increase the price; restrict the availability; make alcohol a national health priority; make alcohol dependence a priority for the National Treatment Agency; stop people binge drinking; save lives on the road; provide alternatives. As one of three authors that contributed to the study *Drug harms in the UK: A multi-criterion decision analysis*, published in the Lancet in 2010[109]

---

[106] M G Griswold et al. *Alcohol use and burden for 195 countries and territories, 1990–2016: a systematic analysis for the Global Burden of Disease Study 2016*, The Lancet https://www.thelancet.com/journals/lancet/article/PIIS0140-6736(18)31310-2/ [17.3.21]

[107] *The Seven Key Messages of the Alcohol Industry*

[108] **David Nutt, *Drugs without the hot air: Making Sense of Legal and Illegal Drugs*,** UIT Cambridge LTD; 2nd edition (16 Jan. 2020)

[109] David Nutt et al. *Drug harms in the UK: a multicriteria decision analysis*, The Lancet, https://www.thelancet.com/journals/lancet/article/PIIS0140-6736(10)61462-6/ [17.3.21]

David is responsible for a very important piece of work that states clearly that alcohol is by far the most harmful widely used recreational drug. Surely it is easy to advise the public that consuming the drug that causes the most harm is something to be avoided. What could be the cause of this bias, and this unwillingness to condemn alcohol as a dangerous, harmful substance that shouldn't be consumed? David owns a wine bar in London and drinks alcohol regularly.

It is comical to think that the highly experienced doctor and author of the study that demonstrated that alcohol causes more harm than all of the other recreational drugs is himself a consumer of alcohol, and the owner of a wine bar. His more recent book *Drink?* further promotes drinking alcohol. He says of alcohol, "you should treat it as more special than eating... Make drinking a positive, active pleasure.. try to reduce how much you are drinking towards the recommended limit while maximising your fun and pleasure." The most harmful drug is harmful because it is poisonous and addictive. It is not fun or pleasurable. The socialising is fun and pleasurable, but we tend to drink alcohol at these social events because we believe it is necessary. David's book is dressed as a scientific study of alcohol but reads like a promotional manual for booze, with positive recommendations on most of its pages: "Being both relaxing and pleasant to take, alcohol encourages habitual use." In fact, alcohol seems relaxing to drinkers but acts as an anesthetic on non-drinkers. It is unpleasant but drinkers put up with the nasty taste and the effect it has on them because it is a highly addictive drug and they feel relief when they drink.

In 2008 the British Medical Association issued *Alcohol misuse: tackling the UK epidemic* which considered "a range of evidence-based policies to tackle the problematic levels of alcohol misuse in the UK" and pointed out that "The vast majority of the UK adult population consume alcohol. The proportion of adults who consume alcohol has been estimated to be 90 per cent in England."[110] This staggering number of drinkers is going to make it very difficult to find any neutral opinions about alcohol. Nine out of 10 adults consume alcohol, so a group of 30 doctors and experts contributing to a study about alcohol harm is likely to be made up of 27 consumers of alcohol. The 650 members of parliament that make up our government are likely to be made up of 585 drinkers. The policy makers and highly educated experts that we trust to write our laws and to ensure society functions as it should are made up of drinkers at a ratio of nine to one. No wonder we have a bias in favour of drinking.

Charity Bias

Drinkaware and Alcohol Change UK are two key charities that inform us about alcohol. Drinkaware has a vested interest in ensuring that we continue to drink alcohol. It describes itself as "an independent charity working to reduce alcohol misuse and harm in the UK," but is funded by the alcohol industry and its ultimate aim is to "change the UK's drinking habits for the better, reduce alcohol-related harm by helping people make better choices about their drinking." Not to stop people drinking, obviously, even though this would be a good way to reduce harm.

Alcohol Change UK was formed from the merger of Alcohol Research UK and Alcohol Concern. It does not accept donations from the alcohol industry but its philosophy is pro-alcohol. Here's what the charity says about alcohol:

> "...in the UK one person every hour dies as a result of alcohol. Alcohol harm – mental health problems, liver disease, one of seven forms of cancer, economic difficulties, and so much more – can affect any one of us, from any walk of life.
>
> We are not anti-alcohol; we are for alcohol change. We are for a future in

---

[110] Charles George et al. *Alcohol misuse: tackling the UK epidemic*, British Medical Association, http://www.dldocs.stir.ac.uk/documents/Alcoholmisuse.pdf [17.3.21]

which people drink as a conscious choice, not a default; where the issues which lead to alcohol problems – like poverty, mental health issues, homelessness – are addressed; where those of us who drink too much, and our loved ones, have access to high-quality support whenever we need it, without shame or stigma.

The problem is complex, and so the solutions aren't simple. But we're ambitious. Driven by our belief that every person deserves to live a full life free from alcohol harm, we create evidence-driven change by working towards five key changes: improved knowledge, better policies and regulation, shifted cultural norms, improved drinking behaviours, and more and better support and treatment."[111]

These three paragraphs are very confusing. The charity recognises that alcohol kills one person every hour but it is not anti-alcohol. Why not? It wants people to drink as a conscious choice. It believes that poverty, mental health issues and homelessness lead to alcohol problems. The charity has its thinking backwards. Alcohol is addictive and it causes its users to develop mental illness, to become homeless and to slip into poverty once they lose their jobs and give up their responsibilities. People don't become homeless and get the sudden urge to have a drink. People don't slide into anxiety, despair and mental illness and then feel the need to drink. Nobody that ended up in poverty suddenly decided they needed to drink because of their situation. Alcohol causes these problems.

The charity says the problem is complex and the solution isn't simple but this is totally wrong. The problem isn't complex and the solution is simple: Don't drink alcohol. Rather than hope that people deserve to live a life free from alcohol harm, they should hope that people live a life free of alcohol. Here's a simple re-write of these three paragraphs: Alcohol kills one person every hour because it is poisonous. The addictive nature of alcohol causes some

---

[111] *About us*, Alcohol Change UK, https://alcoholchange.org.uk/about-us [17.3.21]

drinkers to become mentally ill, homeless and in poverty. Nobody should consume it.

I am sure this charity is staffed by people with noble ambitions but they are clearly drinkers that feel that they are in control of their drinking. How else could a well meaning collection of bright minds manage to miss the obvious fact that alcohol is a dangerous addictive drug that causes death and despair. This charity, that aims to help people affected by alcohol, could make its messaging much clearer and explain why people shouldn't drink. Its work contributes significantly to the public understanding of alcohol consumption but is backed up by a number of other agencies that repeat the same nonsense.

I asked Alcohol Change UK via an enquiry to its press team and a Freedom of Information Request, about the senior team listed on its website, "Could you please confirm that all are drinkers, and let me know if any of them would describe themselves as non-drinkers?" I received a response from Maddy Lawson, Head of Communications: "Our staff make personal choices about their drinking, just as we all do. Some of our staff drink alcohol while others, including members of our senior team, don't drink alcohol and would consider themselves non-drinkers."

Bias - NICE

NICE's major study *Alcohol dependence and harmful alcohol use* is a 613 page document that provides a "guideline on diagnosis, assessment and management of harmful drinking and alcohol dependence." It was last updated in 2020. This is really the bible of understanding how alcohol negatively affects those who suffer harm. 30 extremely knowledgeable professionals were involved in writing the guidance, from professors to doctors, researchers and psychologists. I expect that all of them are drinkers so I asked the press office at NICE if they could tell me. I asked, "how many of the 30 individuals that contributed to this guidance describe themselves as non-drinkers?" Matthew Brown, DIgital Media Manager for NICE, responded to tell me that "this information is not held by NICE." So NICE does not know how many of the contributors are drinkers, and the guidance does not include a disclaimer about whether or not they drink alcohol. It would be helpful if the guidance included a declaration of any interests that could cause the research to be biased.

The report's first sentence already shows bias: "This guideline is concerned with the identification, assessment and management of alcohol dependence and harmful alcohol use." The authors have set out their belief that some drinking should not be classed as dependence, and some alcohol should not be classed as harmful. Their own, obviously. Ask a drinker how much of their use of alcohol is harmful and the result of the addictive properties of alcohol and of course they will say none. They believe they are completely in control.

It continues:

> "However, a growing number of people experience physical, social and psychological harmful effects of alcohol. Twenty-four per cent of the adult population in England, including 33% of men and 16% of women, consumes alcohol in a way that is potentially or actually harmful to their health or well-being (McManus et al., 2009). Four per cent of adults in England are alcohol dependent (6% men; 2% women), which involves a significant degree of addiction to alcohol, making it difficult for them to reduce their drinking or abstain despite increasingly serious harm (Drummond et al., 2005). Alcohol dependence and harmful alcohol use are recognised as mental health disorders by the World Health Organization (WHO, 1992; see Section 2.2). Although not an official diagnostic term, 'alcohol misuse' will be used as a collective term to encompass alcohol dependence and harmful alcohol use throughout this guideline."[112]

---

[112] *Alcohol use disorders*, NICE, https://www.nice.org.uk/guidance/cg115/documents/alcohol-dependence-and-harmful-alcohol-use-full-guideline2 [17.3.21]

This text repeats the myth that there are those in control (the authors obviously) of their drinking but "Twenty-four per cent of the adult population... consumes alcohol in a way that is potentially or actually harmful to their health or well-being." Because alcohol is addictive and toxic, all use of alcohol is harmful. "Four per cent of adults in England are alcohol dependent" is a major misunderstanding. All drinkers are alcohol dependent. They all feel they need it to socialise, they all feel they need to drink wine with dinner. All use of an addictive drug is dependency. If we apply this thinking to the other addictive drugs that sell in huge numbers the same statements sound ridiculous. Would it be credible to say that a small percentage of heroin users are dependent, but that the rest don't have a problem? Or that a small percentage of smokers cause themselves harm, but that the rest are fine? No, all use of addictive drugs is detrimental to their users. Should we categorise users of crack cocaine into two groups, the ones who are dependent on it, and the ones that manage their use? No. Crack is a very addictive form of cocaine, so all use is problematic.

The report also says, "Alcohol dependence and harmful alcohol use are recognised as mental health disorders," which implies wrongly that drinking is the result of mental illness. It is no surprise that repeatedly drinking a toxic chemical, that even the chemical industry describes as dangerous, and that kills germs and santises hospitals, can cause mental illness. Drinkers that repeatedly poison themselves are permanently anxious, their sleep is poor and the toxic chemical causes them further physical and mental harm. The myth that people suffering from mental illness are driven to drink has come about because the people that diagnose them are drinkers. Psychologists, psychiatrists and other mental health professionals like to drink fine wine and they believe they are in control of their drinking. When they see patients who are problem drinking and suffering from mental illness it becomes very difficult to blame the same substance they drink every night. It is much easier to blame the mental illness, rather than to see alcohol as the cause.

The report defines the term, "alcohol misuse" as a "collective term to encompass alcohol dependence and harmful alcohol use." This is one of many examples of the distinction between us and them. Normal drinkers and problem drinkers. It says that alcohol use is fine but alcohol misuse is a problem. All alcohol use produces dependence because it is addictive but the 30 contributing authors of the guidance do not like to accept this. All alcohol use is harmful, and every drinker knows this but they don't like to believe that the posh wine they consume is the same substance that is blighting the mentally ill, homeless, troubled clients they treat.

NICE's accompanying public health guidance entitled *Alcohol-use disorders: prevention*, aims to, "prevent and identify such problems as early as possible using a mix of policy and practice."[113] and is interested in "prevention and early identification of alcohol-use disorders among adults and adolescents." Once again, the use of the phrase "alcohol-use disorder" implies there is normal alcohol use, and abnormal alcohol use, considered a disorder. The guidance recommends that all government agencies interested in public health approach reducing alcohol harm in a coordinated way and has seven recommendations: making alcohol less affordable; making it less easy to buy alcohol; strengthening the current regulations on alcohol marketing; work to improve licencing; allocate resources for screening and brief interventions; support children and young people; screen young people. Nowhere in this guidance is the suggestion that the NHS, or the Department of Health and Social Care, or the Chief Medical Officer, or any other agency that has an interest in protecting the public should tell us not to drink alcohol.

The NICE guidance *Alcohol-use disorders: prevention* exists to inform policy decisions within Government, and these policies in turn will affect the health and wellbeing of the nation. On page 11 are a list of organisations that NICE believes should be consulted on these policy changes, including, "advertisers,

---

[113] *Alcohol-use disorders: prevention,* National Institute for Health and Care Excellence, https://www.nice.org.uk/guidance/ph24/resources/alcoholuse-disorders-prevention-pdf-1996237007557 [17.3.21]

alcohol producers and off- and on-sale retailers."[114] The Government is being advised to set policies in consultation with the alcohol industry. This surely is a serious conflict of interest and will guarantee that the policies are more favourable towards consumption of alcohol. Imagine reading NICE's guidance about tobacco and discovering that they recommended consulting with the tobacco producers. The alcohol industry makes huge profits selling a toxic addictive drug, they should not be involved in policy decisions about that drug.

Putting this in very simple terms, the NICE guidance that informs the nation's public health does not say we shouldn't consume alcohol and reinforces the idea that normal drinking is fine. It also believes that the massively profitable alcohol industry that sells us the addictive poison that damages our health and kills thousands every year, should be involved in the process by which the Chief Medical Officer and the Department of Health create policies. No wonder the nation can't control its drinking!

Compare the guidance on alcohol to NICE's guidance on tobacco. *Stop smoking interventions and services* sets out the latest thinking on smoking using very clear and unambiguous language: "This guideline... aims to ensure that everyone who smokes is advised and encouraged to stop and given the support they need."[115] The language in the guidance doesn't convey the idea that there are two groups of smokers, problem smokers and normal smokers. It doesn't talk about tobacco misuse, or tobacco use disorder. It recognises that all use of tobacco is a problem because tobacco is an addictive poisonous drug. It doesn't look for ways of reducing tobacco use, it says very clearly that people should be advised and encouraged to stop. It also does not recommend that tobacco companies are involved in setting government policy.

---

[114] *Alcohol-use disorders: prevention*, NICE

[115] *Stop smoking interventions and services,* National Institute for Health and Care Excellence, https://www.nice.org.uk/guidance/ng92/resources/stop-smoking-interventions-and-services-pdf-1837751801029 [17.3.21]

NICE issues guidance to keep us safe. Its guidance on tobacco says clearly that smokers should stop smoking, but its guidance about alcohol says we should drink. Both substances are addictive drugs that cause harm and kill their users but because the alcohol guidance is compiled by drinkers it is biased.

In 2007 The Guardian reported on a study by Researchers from the North West Public Health Observatory, at Liverpool John Moores University:

"The true scale of affluent, middle-class drinking is revealed today with the publication of figures showing that more than a quarter of adults living in some of the wealthiest towns, such as Harrogate and Guildford, are drinking enough alcohol every week to damage their health.

The figures, commissioned by the government, show a north-south divide, with heavy, steady drinking highest in the Surrey commuter belt.. The breakdown of drinking statistics for every local authority was requested by the government, which for the first time this year pointed the finger at the middle-class, middle-aged habitual wine-drinker."

The public health minister, Dawn Primarolo, yesterday made it clear the government felt it was time to move on from the battle to clear the streets of binge-drinking youths and tackle the drinking culture hidden behind the sitting room curtains.

"We need to be clear the figures are for all alcohol-related hospital admissions, not casualty figures. Most of these are not young people, they are 'everyday' drinkers who have drunk too much for too long. This has to change," she said.

The figures show a substantial amount of hazardous drinking across England, hitherto largely ignored because it does not happen on the streets."[116]

This story is rare. A truthful look at where the harm from alcohol is happening. Middle class drinkers that think they are in control drinking wine every night in the suburbs. It's not as visible as the problem drinking that we see on the streets but this is where alcohol does the damage - regular use by people who believe that alcohol is benign and do not believe that it is a harmful, addictive drug. Drinkers buy in to the marketing about wine and spirits as sophisticated products that convey status and wealth, their use increases over time because it is addictive, and they are harmed as a result of the toxicity.

David Nutt reluctantly points out the same thing, quoting a study by the UK's leading alcohol and liver disease expert, Professor Nick Sheron, "a third of patients with severe alcohol-induced liver damage had never even considered that they were drinking abnormally." He is right to highlight the fact that drinkers that feel their intake is normal can cause themselves damage. Again though, this is the voice of an expert making a distinction between normal drinking and abnormal drinking. These individuals were drinking normally and it caused them liver damage. Drinking a toxic substance night after night causes damage. He goes on to say, "only 9 percent showed evidence of severe alcohol dependence."[117] So 81% are considered to not be dependent on alcohol but damage their liver anyway. Regular drinking that leads to liver damage is alcohol dependence. All drinking is alcohol dependence.

All the guidance and messaging that is available to drinkers fails to tell them not to drink it, and reinforces the fact that it is fine in moderation. Imagine if we were told that smoking cigarettes is fine in moderation. Cigarettes are addictive and poisonous, damaging the lungs and causing cancer. We are told

---

[116] Sarah Boseley, *Scale of harmful middle class drinking revealed*, The Guardian, https://www.theguardian.com/society/2007/oct/16/drugsandalcohol.health [17.3.21]

[117] *Drink?*, David Nutt

to stop smoking and we see the warnings on the side of cigarette packets. If you smoke some cigarettes you will be a smoker, and smoking is dangerous. If we were told by the government that some heroin use is misuse but that it is fine in moderation, we would see an increase in heroin use. Like alcohol, some heroin use will lead to more heroin use. An addictive drug will lead its users to consume it again and again, and in the case of alcohol, to consume it more and more. The result of the guidance is that people continue to drink, and end up drinking more, and they cause themselves harm.

Bias - The NHS

The NHS plays a major part in the widespread unhelpful guidance about alcohol. Here is the text from its website about drinking:

> "To keep health risks from alcohol to a low level if you drink most weeks:
>
> - men and women are advised not to drink more than 14 units a week on a regular basis
>
> - spread your drinking over 3 or more days if you regularly drink as much as 14 units a week
>
> - if you want to cut down, try to have several drink-free days each week
>
> - Fourteen units is equivalent to 6 pints of average-strength beer or 10 small glasses of low-strength wine."[118]

This guidance about units is so simple and the NHS is highly trusted so it is no surprise that the advice has become part of the way we talk about and think about alcohol. The idea of limiting the number of units that we all drink is ingrained in the minds of all drinkers. This guidance is written in simple and clear language and is easily understood but it seriously misunderstands the addictive properties of alcohol. For the occasional drinker the guidance appears to be sensible - we each should try to limit our intake. But because

---

[118] *The risks of drinking too much*, NHS, https://www.nhs.uk/live-well/alcohol-support/the-risks-of-drinking-too-much [17.3.21]

alcohol is addictive, every drinker will tend towards consuming more alcohol. So regular drinkers will become more regular drinkers. Binge drinkers will drink more every time. Alcohol is addictive, and becomes more addictive the more we drink.

The NHS has the authority and evidence to be able to state quite clearly that all alcohol use is harmful, that drinking alcohol will lead to an increasing level of drinking, that it causes cancer, that it causes harm. The NHS is the institution that we trust to look after us. Our national health is in its hands. It would be much more helpful to provide simple guidance that keeps us safe from harm - don't drink alcohol. The title of the NHS's site is *The risks of drinking too much*, which again is another example of biased thinking. It could be more accurately titled *The risks of drinking*.

At each A&E department and in every hospital there are NHS doctors, nurses and support staff that see the effects of alcohol on the public. From cancer to brain damage, to liver problems, to cirrhosis, to head injuries, to pancreatic problems to accidents and falls. All NHS staff are affected by the harm caused by alcohol. They see injured patients and drinkers from all strata of society that have harmed themselves by drinking. From an article in the Guardian entitled *Chaotic lives and ethical dilemmas: inside the hospital liver ward* is an overview of what NHS staff see every day:

> *"John smiles weakly again and says: "Well, well." It's a good day though. Asked again where he is, five minutes later, John gets it right. Tomorrow he will probably be mystified by the question again. He is 52 and has Korsakoff's syndrome, a form of dementia brought on by his drinking. Alcohol has damaged his brain as well as his liver and it's permanent...*

> *I can only ever drink two glasses of wine and then I'm drunk," she says... "I did used to drink a lot, especially when I was going through my divorce. Just wine," she says... Yet Rita, who worked as a PA until April last year, has yellow jaundiced skin caused by alcoholic liver disease and cirrhosis.*

Last week it all seemed so hopeful. "We went out for a meal on Sunday – the three of us," he says. Then on Tuesday he woke up bleeding from the stomach and was rushed to hospital. He knows his only chance now is to stop completely.

Len, who drinks eight cans of strong lager a day, is emaciated, with a tendency to wave his hands in the air as he speaks. He is 52 but looks 20 years older and has end-stage liver disease."[119]

The British Medical Association's report *Reducing alcohol-related harm: a blueprint for Government* says, "Doctors witness these harms in their everyday working lives. In England in 2016, there were over 5,500 alcohol-specific deaths and over 1.1 million alcohol-related hospital admissions, while there is a well-established association between alcohol and violence (in 40% of violent incidents, victims perceived the offender to be under the influence of alcohol).3 As well as the health harms, there are significant economic and societal costs - alcohol is estimated to cost £21 billion a year in England, including £3.5 billion a year to the NHS (2009-10 costs)."[120]

These figures show that the impact of our alcohol consumption is massive and costly, including £3.5 billion of direct cost to the NHS in 2010. These huge numbers are evidence that the NHS's guidance is ineffective. Every drinker that tries to moderate their drinking will find it difficult. Alcohol is addictive, and drinking alcohol causes it to become more addictive. The NHS staff members on the frontline see the damage it causes but the powers that be continue the mistaken approach, that moderation is the solution. The report issued by the British Medical Association aims to reduce the harm caused by alcohol and provides recommendations for the government. Of course, not

---

[119] Sarah Boseley, *Chaotic lives and ethical dilemmas: inside the hospital liver ward*, The Guardian, https://www.theguardian.com/society/2016/jan/24/inside-the-liver-ward-nhs [17.3.21]

[120] *Reducing alcohol-related harm: a blueprint for Government*, British Medical Association, https://www.bma.org.uk/media/2072/tackling-alcohol-related-harm-in-england.pdf [17.3.21]

one of these recommendations is to tell the public to stop drinking.

The guidance on alcohol units is ultimately the responsibility of the Chief Medical Officers in the UK. The government website says, "the Chief Medical Officer (CMO) acts as the UK government's principal medical adviser, and the professional head of all directors of public health in local government and the medical profession in government... The CMO provides public health and clinical advice to ministers in the Department of Health and Social Care (DHSC) and across government... The CMO is supported by 3 Deputy Chief Medical Officers."[121] Ideally these individuals would be non-drinkers, and therefore have no bias towards consuming alcohol.

The BMJ, the NHS, NICE and the DHSC all work together to write guidance to keep us safe. Each one of these agencies is happy to tell us that alcohol is harmful but none of them is able to tell us not to drink it. It shouldn't be a surprise that the guidance is biased because the majority of the individuals that contributed to the guidance are drinkers. I don't listen to advice about smoking from smokers, I wouldn't accept advice from opiate users about the drug they take and I don't believe advice about cocaine from cocaine users. The government gives us advice about alcohol that encourages us to drink, written by drinkers. This is dangerous and misguided. If you want the truth about alcohol try to seek out guidance written by non-drinkers.

---

[121] *Chief Medical Officer and DHSC Chief Scientific Adviser* **Professor Chris Whitty**, https://www.gov.uk/government/people/christopher-whitty [17.3.21]

23

Beliefs

Addiction is a combination of two things: a drug (or activity) that causes a chemical change in the user and a belief that there is a benefit to using the drug. There is no way to change the effect of the drug but it is relatively straightforward to change the things that users believe about the drug. I met a fit and healthy 50 year old on holiday recently who didn't drink. When I asked him why not he said he drank a pint of lager once when he was about 18 after his mates convinced him he should become a drinker like them. He said he didn't like the taste and it made him feel unsteady so he never drank alcohol again. Lucky man. He tried alcohol and didn't like the taste or the effect, which is true of all of us when we first try alcohol, but more importantly he refused to adopt the beliefs of the friends that introduced him to alcohol.

Below are the beliefs that drinkers cling onto, compared to the beliefs that non-drinkers maintain. Any drinker that can switch their thinking, giving up the mistaken beliefs and accepting the truth, should find it easy to give up alcohol.

- Drinkers believe that alcohol tastes nice. Non drinkers believe that alcohol tastes foul. If in doubt, give it to a child to try. Remember that we found it unpleasant when we first tried it. It is formed when fruit and grain rots. It is a poisonous chemical used to sanitise and kill germs.

- Drinkers believe that alcohol is relaxing. Non-drinkers know that relaxation comes from tasks completed, and work well done. Alcohol gets in the way of getting things done. It appears to relax drinkers but this is relief from the need for a drink. Alcohol is not relaxing to non-drinkers, it is an anesthetic.

- Drinkers believe that alcohol de-stresses. Non-drinkers know that alcohol does not relieve stress, it is an anesthetic. In fact, alcohol causes anxiety. Drinking alcohol adds stress and prevents drinkers getting things done. Hangovers are characterised by lethargy and anxiety. Alcohol interferes with sleep and can lead to mental illness.

- Drinkers believe that alcohol is a key part of the social scene. Non-drinkers know that alcohol impedes good conversation and causes people to be boring and repetitive, to lose their judgement, to lose control of their emotions. We are perfect social beings in our natural state.

- Drinkers believe that alcohol is sophisticated. Non-drinkers don't buy into this. Alcohol is sold to us as sophisticated but we don't have to believe it. Drinkers become much less sophisticated when they consume it. The drinks industry has tricked drinkers. Alcohol is a toxic, harmful, drug.

- Drinkers believe that alcohol is pleasurable. Non-drinkers know there is natural pleasure in seeing friends, eating nice food, parties and social events. Drinkers confuse drinking at these occasions with the natural positive experience. The occasion is the pleasure, not the alcohol. Alcohol is an unpleasant anesthetic - try it out of context to experience it.

- Drinkers believe that alcohol makes them less shy and/or more confident. Non-drinkers know that shyness is normal. We all take time to warm up in a new social situation. Alcohol interferes with our judgement and makes us overly loud and obnoxious. It does not build confidence. Confidence increases and shyness dissipates when we socialise without alcohol.

· Drinkers believe that drinking alcohol is a free choice. In fact alcohol is highly addictive. One drink makes the drinker want to drink again. Alcohol causes the brain to produce stress hormones and this causes anxiety, which the next drink relieves.

· Drinkers believe that they would be deprived if they couldn't drink alcohol. Non-drinkers don't experience this. Giving up alcohol will make drinkers happier, more in control, healthier, with more time and more money. A drinker that becomes a non-drinker will feel a new freedom.

· Drinkers believe that alcohol consumption is natural and normal. Non-drinkers are not deficient in any way. Nature made us perfect. Each human is amazing at socialising, communicating and interaction. Our systems and controls keep us safe from harm. Alcohol is detrimental to us. We should reject it.

One of the key beliefs that keeps drinkers consuming alcohol is that certain situations and activities cannot be enjoyed without a drink. Parties, the pub, dinner in a restaurant, weddings, etc. These activities are great without alcohol but the drinker feels deprived if they can't drink. Being deprived of alcohol is a powerful state of mind and although there is a physical aspect to the addictive properties of alcohol, the state of being deprived of something that appears essential to an enjoyable evening is very powerful. When the desire is satisfied, and the deprived drinker is finally able to have a drink, the sense of relief is also very powerful, and this moment of a restriction being lifted, again reinforces the belief that the alcohol provides a benefit.

A number of diets are based on the philosophy that the individual must not consume something that they find pleasurable. As an example, cake is nice but we can't eat it when we are on a diet. This makes the cake become a desirable item, and the thought of eating cake becomes more desirable because of the unattainable nature of the cake. The dieter may find the forbidden cake lodges in the mind, and the more they are restricted from eating the forbidden cake the more desirable the cake becomes.

Almost every treatment aimed at individuals struggling with addiction has the same philosophy, accepting that alcohol is pleasurable and desirable. In turn they advise the client not to drink the desirable alcohol, and this restriction makes the unattainable drink seem even more desirable. The poor drinker in the pub, restaurant or party cannot relax and enjoy themselves because the thing they must not consume becomes ever more desirable. Their belief that the enjoyment of the experience is in some way down to the alcohol they consume, has caused them to believe that the evening now cannot be enjoyed without the alcohol. Any approach to treating addiction that does not tackle the desirability of alcohol will not work, and has the effect of making the alcohol even more desired.

The method that does work is to change the beliefs of the drinker about alcohol to ensure that the desire for the alcohol is switched off in the drinker. This change of beliefs leads to a lifetime free of alcohol, and is easy to achieve. Provided the ex-drinker maintains the new beliefs in the face of the peer pressure they will experience from other drinkers, they will be free of alcohol for life without feeling deprived. Remember none of us believed that we needed to drink alcohol at parties, or that we couldn't enjoy dinner without wine, when we were children. Other drinkers convinced us, and the alcohol industry welcomed us with falsehoods about the product they sold us. We were easily convinced that alcohol is necessary, and we can be easily convinced that alcohol is not just unnecessary, but detrimental.

24

Trauma and pain

I have a trick question that I like to ask drinkers. What is the cause of addiction to alcohol? The answer obviously, is alcohol. Because it is an addictive drug, drinkers will drink more of it, and drink it more often. When I ask drinkers that question though, the range of typical answers is surprising. Trauma, childhood issues, emotional pain, upheaval, depression, homelessness and mental illness feature heavily. The belief that pain and trauma are the cause of problem drinking is widespread, and pervasive among experts. Addiction practitioners, scientists and medical professionals highlight trauma, poverty, and social problems that lead people to be addicted to substances. Here is Dr Ben Sessa, an addiction psychiatrist and senior research fellow at Imperial College London who conducted a study using MDMA to get heavy drinkers to stop drinking, explaining to the Guardian newspaper: "most addiction is based on underlying trauma, often from childhood."[122] This view is a sweeping generalisation and is not borne out by evidence. It is true that some people that suffer trauma drink too much but there are plenty of heavy drinkers that have never suffered childhood trauma, and plenty of people that have suffered trauma that don't drink.

---

[122] Helena Blackstone, *MDMA treatment for alcoholism could reduce relapse, study suggests*, The Guardian, https://www.theguardian.com/society/2019/aug/19/mdma-treatment-alcoholism-relapse-study [17.3.21]

The Priory is one of the more famous treatment centres for individuals suffering from addiction. Here is some text from its website:

> *"Research indicates that it is likely that there are a number of contribut-ing factors that can lead you to develop an addiction to alcohol... which can be both genetic and environmental in nature... Research suggests that you are at increased risk of developing alcohol addiction if you have a close family member with an addiction, such as a parent or sibling... If you are already struggling with an untreated mental health condition such as anxiety or depression, you may be at greater risk of developing alcohol addiction... Stressful life events such as bereavement, losing a job, experiencing a traumatic event or struggling with financial problems, have also been linked to the development of alcohol addiction."*[123]

It would be helpful if the website told the truth. Alcohol is the common factor that causes people to become addicted to alcohol. In the same way that nicotine is the factor that causes people to smoke. There may be some people who are depressed and drink too much, some going through difficult times that drink too much, and some who grew up in a drinking family that drink too much, but there are also plenty of people in exactly the same situation that decide not to drink. It must be worrying for the normal well adjusted, comfortable individual, that has a job, a family, a home and a normal life who decides to seek help from the Priory. A drinker that feels they don't have a genetic factor, a mental health condition or are going through a difficult situation would struggle to find something in the Priory's text that seems to fit their situation. What about the normal, everyday drinker?

A story in the Guardian entitled *Women, The Hidden Risks of Drinking*, demon-strates that there are widespread alcohol-related health problems among all social classes irrespective of background, and that regular consumption of

---

[123] *What are the causes of alcoholism?* The Priory, https://www.priorygroup.com/addiction-treatment/alcohol-rehab/causes-of-alcoholism [17.3.21]

wine among the middle classes is causing a surge in health problems. The story shares the experience of Dr Gray Smith-Laing of the Medway Maritime Hospital in Kent: "Many of his patients have been drinking excessively for years. 'These are the steady drinkers. Typically they have a half-bottle of wine with their meal every night, or at lunchtime, and another drink at dinner. They are never drunk but they drink in a sustained manner. They don't realise they've got a problem because they think alcoholics are down-and-outs, or pub regulars. They have wine with their meal and because of that they somehow think that takes away the harm, or they say, "but I don't drink spirits". These misconceptions are very common... 'Any liver specialist would tell the same story,' adds Smith-Laing grimly. 'Alcohol is a totally classless disease. It may be more discreet among the upper and middle classes, because they do a lot of it at home. But it causes harm across all social classes.'"[124]

Drinkers aren't comfortable with recognising that the substance they consume is an addictive drug. We are all sold the lie that our drinks are sophisticated and show that we have good taste and refinement and all drinkers believe that the decision to drink alcohol is a free choice. Drinkers will blame anything but the alcohol for the problems that they see other drinkers afflicted by. They prefer to believe that mental illness leads to drink, that homeless people turn to the bottle, and that the drinkers in A&E and hospital wards have suffered something in their past that caused them to harm themselves. Because the reality is too unpleasant to contemplate - that ordinary people like them, drinking much the same alcohol, have ended up giving up their responsibilities, losing their money, suffering harm and losing control of their mental faculties.

Drinkers are affected by a number of factors that may have an impact on their drinking, for example availability, pricing and their own personal circumstances. In Sweden, all alcohol over 3.5% is sold by the Swedish

---

[124] Denis Campbell, *Women: the hidden risks of drinking*, The Guardian, https://www.theguardian.com/society/2008/feb/24/drugsandalcohol.health1 [17.3.21]

Government's Systembolaget shops, which close at 3.00pm on a Saturday and stay closed for the rest of the weekend. Swedish drinkers that finish their last bottle of wine at 9.00pm on Saturday night can't pop out to the local shop to buy more. Sweden also taxes its alcohol more highly than the UK and the higher prices reduce demand. As a result, UK drinking levels are higher than Sweden's at around 11 litres per person annually in the UK versus 8 litres per person in Sweden.[125] Would an expert blame the increased intake among the UK population versus Sweden on higher levels of trauma? Are the public in the UK more likely to have a genetic disposition to drink? No, it's just cheaper and more available here. Alcohol Change UK points out that in the UK, "The North East, North West and South West have higher levels of consumption than London and the South East, for example. In Scotland, consumption levels are consistently higher than in England, with most of the difference being accounted for by cheap alcohol sold in off-licences."[126]

The gin craze of the late 17th century in the UK is an example of how an increase in the availability of alcohol can result in public harm. King William III came to the throne in 1689 and started a trade war with France. He implemented heavy tax on wine and cognac entering the UK. This caused them to be more expensive resulting in reduced demand. At the same time, The Corn Laws in England provided tax breaks on the production of spirits, resulting in a massive expansion of strong alcohol in England. The gin craze emerged as a result of the new fashionable and extremely potent alcohol. Rich and poor people alike drank it with wild abandon and it was often sold by enterprising stalls and pop-ups, for example offering hot gin and gingerbread in winter.

Five years later and with mounting levels of insanity and death among the

---

[125] *UK comparisons with other countries*, Drinkaware,
    https://www.drinkaware.co.uk/research/research-and-evaluation-reports/
    comparisons [17.3.21]

[126] *Drinking trends in the UK*, Alcohol Change UK https://alcoholchange.org.uk/alcohol-facts/
    fact-sheets/drinking-trends-in-the-uk [17.3.21]

gin fuelled public, a distiller's license was introduced at £50, a huge sum. This stopped the expansion of distillers but didn't stop the problem. William Hogarth's famous etching of Gin Lane showed people of the era losing their minds to gin: a negligent mother, a self harming drunk man, a suicidal barber and a widespread syphilis problem. Gin's ubiquitous availability and very low price led to widespread death, insanity, negligence and poverty. The Gin Act of 1751 raised taxes and fees for retailers and made licenses more difficult to come by, which finally began to reduce consumption.

The gin craze is a perfect illustration of the cause of problem drinking. Gin, like every alcoholic drink, is harmful and addictive. If an addictive drug is suddenly readily available and very cheap then it is natural to expect consumption to rise. The increase in consumption of a harmful drug will lead to an increase in mental health problems, homelessness, physical harm, and death rates. Compare the thinking of the so called experts that believe that childhood trauma or family upbringing is the cause of problem drinking. The gin craze wasn't the result of a sudden increase in childhood trauma. Gin didn't suddenly become popular because the public was brought up in a drinking household. Alcohol is addictive, and to those that drink it, suddenly lowering the price or increasing the availability, will allow them to drink more.

25

Genetics and an addictive personality

There is a common belief that some people are likely to be addicted to a drug because of some aspect of their character or their genetics. Maybe they have an addictive personality or they came from a drinking household and are more likely to drink. Maybe they have a gene that means they are more likely to be addicts. These ideas are much more prevalent in the studies and commentary about drinking alcohol and much less prevalent in the thinking about other addictive drugs, and this is the result in the bias inherent in the studies and work that has been developed by drinkers. Our thinking about smoking is a good example. Smokers start smoking for one reason only, because other smokers convinced them to, and they continue to smoke because nicotine is addictive. Nobody picked up a cigarette, or continues to smoke because they have an addictive personality or because of something in their genes. Advice to smokers says stop smoking and identifies nicotine as the cause of the addiction. Don't smoke, because cigarettes are highly addictive and harmful. There are very few studies that search for a reason why people smoke cigarettes because it is accepted that nicotine is addictive, and the obvious solution is to stop smoking.

Drinking alcohol has similarities with smoking tobacco – both are harmful addictive drugs – but the theories and studies about our alcohol intake miss the obvious fact that alcohol is addictive. Imagine if using a search engine to type in, "why do people get addicted to alcohol?" and getting the result, "because alcohol is addictive." There would be no need to plough through pages of nonsense because we'd already have our answer. This truth is simple and basic and if we all believed it, we wouldn't need to plough millions of dollars into research and complicated studies. Unfortunately the drinkers that feel they are in control of their drinking don't like the answer and refuse to believe the truth.

Nobody had an urge to have their first drink because of their personality or genes. Each person started drinking because they were encouraged to drink by other drinkers. And because alcohol is addictive, every drinker that continues to drink, will tend to drink more.

There are a number of factors that have an influence on the drinker's intake, including their lifestyle, their circle of friends, family, hobbies and responsibilities. Alcohol Change UK says, "Compared to other children, children of parents who are alcohol dependent are... four times more likely to become dependent drinkers themselves." and this makes a lot of sense but is likely to not be genetic, but the result of various factors. Growing up in a house where wine is consumed with every meal for example may normalise the drinking of wine with meals. If a drinker's first drinking experience was provided by their parents it may be more embedded in the drinker's beliefs that it is a part of normal life to consume alcohol. There is anecdotal evidence that if the person that introduced a smoker to cigarettes was seen as cool or interesting in some way, the smoker will find it more difficult to break their addiction to nicotine. In the same way, if a parent introduces a child to alcohol consumption this may be more influential than if the drinker's peers encouraged the first drinking experience.

Reviewing the massive number of studies on addiction and genetics produces so many conflicting and nuanced results that it is nigh on impossible to say in simple terms how tiny differences in our genes makes us more or less likely to find a specific substance addictive. The study *Genetics of cocaine and methamphetamine consumption and preference* published by the non-profit PLOS says simply, "it remains challenging to determine genetic risk factors for substance abuse in human populations."[127] The study, *Genetics and alcoholism* reported: "It should be emphasized that while genetic differences affect risk, there is no "gene for alcoholism," and both environmental and social factors weigh heavily on the outcome."[128] These two quotes are simple and basic and discount the theory that alcohol addiction is the result of genetics. The American Addiction Centres Alcohol.org website says, "there are few long-term studies that have conclusively linked specific genetic traits to humans who struggle with AUD [Alcohol Use Disorder]."[129]

Differences in genes do have an impact in the way that we respond to alcohol but these are subtle and affect our immediate response rather than our propensity for addiction. Here's an example of these subtle differences, discovered by geneticists and researchers, from the University of Pennsylvania School of Medicine quoted in Science News:

> "The researchers identified 13 independent genetic variants associated with alcohol consumption, eight of which had not been previously reported, including VRK2, DCLK2, ISL1, FTO, IGF2BP1, PPR1R3B, BRAP, and RBX1. Ten variants were associated with AUD, including seven that had not been previously associated with it: GCKR, SIX3, SLC39A8, DRD2 (rs4936277 and rs61902812), chr10q25.1, and FTO. The five variants associated with both heavy drinking and AUD were ADH1B, ADH1C, FTO,

---

[127] Chad Highfill et al. *Genetics of cocaine and methamphetamine consumption and preference in Drosophila melanogaster*, PLOS Genetics,
https://journals.plos.org/plosgenetics/article?id=10.1371/journal.pgen.1007834
[17.3.21]

[128] Howard Edenberg and Tatiana Foroud, *Genetics and alcoholism*, National Center for Biotechnology Information, U.S. National Library of Medicine,
https://www.ncbi.nlm.nih.gov/pmc/articles/PMC4056340/ [17.3.21]

[129] *Is Alcoholism Inherited?* American Addiction Centers, https://www.alcohol.org/alcoholism/is-it-inherited/ [17.3.21]

GCKR, and SLC39A8.

*They also discovered 188 different genetic correlations to health out-
comes among the study group, some in opposite directions. Notably,
heavy drinking was associated with lower risk of coronary artery disease
and glycemic traits, including type 2 diabetes, but positively correlated
with overall health rating, HDL or "good" cholesterol concentration,
and years of education. AUD [Alcohol Use Disorder] was significantly
correlated with 111 traits or diseases, including lower intelligence and
likelihood of quitting smoking and greater risk of insomnia and most
psychiatric disorders. The genetic differences between the two alcohol-
related conditions and the observed opposite correlations point to
potentially important differences in comorbidity and prognosis. That
underscores the need to identify the effects of the risk variants in future,
especially where they diverge by traits, to better understand and treat
them, the authors said."*[130]

This confusing outcome, of 188 different genetic correlations, may be relevant
to scientists, geneticists and researchers but it is so complex that it doesn't
help any less-scientifically minded members of the public who want to
understand the addictive properties of alcohol. It is irrelevant to drinkers who
have found that their drinking levels have escalated to the point where their
intake is a problem. Alcohol may produce subtly different reactions in each of
us but the simple fact is that it is addictive to those that drink it. For anyone
who finds that their consumption has become a problem the easiest advice
would be to stop drinking it. Searching for intricate and detailed scientific
findings is the calling of scientists, and finding subtle variations in our genes
is the calling of geneticists. Drinkers need to understand the basics of alcohol.

Many of the studies reviewing how our genes produce variants in the way
alcohol affects us end with the conclusion that more research is required,

---

[130] *Study reveals genes associated with heavy drinking and alcoholism,* Science Daily,
https://www.sciencedaily.com/releases/2019/04/190402124314.htm [17.3.21]

or that further study is necessary. Studies lead to more studies, and the findings are not conclusive. The study quoted above concludes, "The genetic differences between the two alcohol-related conditions and the observed opposite correlations point to potentially important differences in comorbidity and prognosis. That underscores the need to identify the effects of the risk variants in future,"[131] which isn't really a conclusion.

Here's another non-conclusion from a study entitled *Overview of the Genetics of Alcohol Use Disorder* published in the Oxford University Press:

"Despite the evidence supporting the prominence of genetic factors in [Alcohol Use Disorder] AUD's etiology, the identification of genetic risk variants has been difficult and labor intensive. With recent advances in technology, the most promising results stem from recent GWAS, which have helped to identify new variants in the genetics of AUD. Among the variants identified, the most significant SNPs remain in the alcohol metabolism enzyme genes, ADH and ALDH. Importantly, the prevalence of the various isoforms of ADH and ALDH differs among ethnicities and populations. Therefore, lower alcohol consumption in certain populations, as a result of the protective effect of alcohol metabolism SNPs, may be due to gene-environment interactions.

AUD prevention could be enhanced with a growing knowledge of the disorder's neurobiology and genetics. A growing body of literature on AUD genetics will improve both the understanding of at-risk individuals' biology and the development of new medications. Although information such as family history can currently be used to identify at-risk individuals, understanding the genetic architecture of AUD could enable us to pinpoint these individuals with greater certainty. Understanding of the genetic risk factors involved could be important to guide personalized treatments of patients who have already developed

---

[131] *Study reveals genes associated with heavy drinking and alcoholism,* Science Daily

AUD and to inform the development of new pharmacological and other novel interventions."[132]

This confusing text is saying that there may be the potential for developing medications, and that we may be able to identify at-risk individuals. The study "has been difficult and labor intensive," but its conclusion is very inconclusive. Wouldn't it be easier to say that we don't need medications to treat people that drink a lot, we should just advise them not to drink. And that the identification of at risk people is simple - drinkers are at risk because alcohol is addictive and harmful.

Common sense and our own experiences provide us with the truth in most areas of our life and allow us to make rational and sensible decisions. Whatever the subtleties and variations present in our specific genetic profile we all share a common experience when we consume alcohol. There are 7 billion humans on the planet, all much the same as each other and we all feel the same effect when we drink a glass of wine. The same dose of the same drug given to a large population would produce much the same effect in all of us. Different factors will have an effect such as the amount of food in the drinker's stomach at the time they drink, or an increased tolerance based on the amount of drinking over time, but these are circumstantial, not genetic, and not the result of our personality.

If we had an opportunity to test a wide cross section of the drinkers that died in 2020 because of their alcohol intake, or we could test a cross section of the down and out city dwellers that have ended up homeless because of their alcohol intake, we would not see a common genetic variant present in each of them. Blonde, blue eyed tall people are just as likely to suffer alcohol harm as short dark people. Individuals from African, Asian or European backgrounds,

---

[132] Elisabeth Tawa et al. *Overview of the Genetics of Alcohol Use Disorder, Alcohol and Alcoholism,* Volume 51, Oxford Academic, https://academic.oup.com/alcalc/article/51/5/507/2237006 [17.3.21]

in terms of their genetic profiles, are equally likely to drink heavily and suffer harm. Our individual reaction may be subtly different but alcohol is addictive to each of us.

The majority of our common drugs work equally well on all humans. Pharmaceuticals such as paracetamol, valium, aspirin, ibuprofen, steroids and antihistamines work when we take them. If we have muscle pain, ibuprofen provides relief. Paracetamol works to reduce the pain of a headache. Aspirin thins the blood. These work for everybody. There is no need to study our genetics to investigate the differences in the way that paracetamol works on us. Scientists don't review our complex reactions to paracetamol and produce findings that show that there are multiple variations in genetic differences that mean that we do or do not find our headaches reducing by a little bit more or a little bit less. Paracetamol is a basic drug. We take it when we have a headache and the pain goes away.

We wouldn't accept the argument that these drugs work differently on people with different personalities. The idea of an addictive personality is repeated regularly when we talk about alcohol. Imagine if we believed that paracetamol works differently on some people because of their personality. Does aspirin thin the blood of people differently if they have a slight variation in their personality? No.

Are there small differences in the way that these drugs work on us because of slight differences in our genes? Possibly. Does it matter? No, because aspirin thins the blood more or less equally in every human being. Paracetamol reduces pain. Ibuprofen reduces muscle inflammation. In the same way, we should think of alcohol in very basic terms because it is a simple drug that works more or less equally on every human being. Studies of why some people are affected differently by alcohol are the result of the same bias and misunderstanding that results from the guidance being written by drinkers.

Our language about drugs and the way they work typically places the drug as the subject in the way we talk about them. For example "paracetamol kills pain" makes paracetamol the subject, having an action, killing pain, acting on a human. "Steroids can help destroy cancer cells and make chemotherapy more effective," is another typical example where we name the drug as the provider of an effect that works on a patient. This basic language is clear and straightforward but is often turned on its head when we talk about alcohol. A sentence about the addictive properties of alcohol would say, "alcohol is addictive," – alcohol is the subject, acting on people that drink it. Because the individuals that write about alcohol are drinkers and they don't like to admit that the drug that they appear to enjoy could be universally addictive they use language that reverses the norm and makes the drinker the subject. We see phraseology such as "who can get addicted to alcohol," or "can I get addicted?", which have the effect of introducing doubt about the universal effect and questioning the property of alcohol.

"We get addicted to alcohol" downgrades the addictive properties of alcohol and blames the individuals. "Alcohol is addictive" focuses on the alcohol as the object. The language shifts the blame. "Sarah is an addict" would be better written as "x is addictive and Sarah uses it." The drug is the addictive object and Sarah is the subject that the drug has acted on. At Alcoholics Anonymous the attendees say, "Hi, I am Charlie, and I am an alcoholic." but this shifts the blame onto the individual, Charlie and away from the addictive substance. "Hi, I am Charlie and alcohol is extremely addictive," would focus the attention where it ought to be focused, on the addictive, harmful substance.

In David Nutt's book *Drink?* David starts the chapter *Addiction: Have I got an alcohol problem*, with the unambiguous statement: "It's not your fault you want to drink. Alcohol is a powerful and addictive drug." This is a good start but then he spends a chapter offering various theories that move the blame for addiction away from alcohol. "Am I becoming dependent?" is an unusual question when it refers to a "powerful and addictive drug" and would be better phrased as "alcohol makes its users dependent."[133] At one point he identifies some traits that can result in alcohol being addictive including: the anxiety that comes from talking to girls (a sexist comment because the author believes that girls don't get nervous talking to boys); having fun; emotional pain. These are very strange ideas. With each of these points David shifts the blame away from alcohol, no surprise because he is a drinker.

Alcohol works on the people that drink it. It is addictive to all drinkers. It becomes more addictive the more that the drinker has consumed but this is because all humans react in the same way by producing increasing levels of cortisol as they consume more. It is better to think of alcohol as a subject that acts on the people that drink it. Questions such as can I get addicted?, who can get addicted?, am I addicted?, cause us to believe that we respond differently to alcohol and miss the obvious truth. Is alcohol addictive? Yes. Like every addictive drug, if we use it, it will have an addictive effect on us. Will each of us end up harmed by it, or homeless or dead? That depends on whether we exercise restraint. It is not dependent on whether we have addictive genes, or an addictive personality.

When drinkers that believe they are in control of their drinking want to understand how some people have lost control of their drinking they will understandably not be keen to blame alcohol and instead will look for other factors. The studies are biased because they are conducted by drinkers and they fail to see the obvious issue hiding in plain sight. The cause of alcohol harm is alcohol and the cause of alcohol addiction is alcohol. There is no genetic difference between someone who has died from drinking too much and someone who drinks one glass of wine every night. The same substance that provides what seems like pleasure to the occasional drinker causes more harm to those that drink more of it. And the addictive properties of alcohol mean that people that drink are likely to drink more of it. The common feature of the homeless population in the big city is that they all drink alcohol.

---

133 David Nutt, *Drink?*

The common feature of all the individuals that died because of their alcohol intake in 2020 is the alcohol they drank. What is the best way of preventing individuals being harmed by alcohol? Tell them not to drink it. The range of studies that examine our genetic differences seem only to produce confusing headlines and detail that does not help the public understand alcohol.

26

Alcoholics Anonymous

Alcoholics Anonymous provides free support through its network of meetings and via a huge community of individuals who have decided not to drink alcohol. The members that meet to support each other in the fellowship have had direct experience of the control that alcohol exerts over the individual and have realised that drinking alcohol is a negative experience. It asks its members to declare at each meeting that they are an alcoholic. Here's how its website defines alcoholism:

> *While there is no formal "AA definition" of alcoholism, the majority of our members agree that, for most of us, it could be described as a physical compulsion, coupled with a mental obsession... As alcoholics, we have learned the hard way that willpower alone, however strong in other respects, was not enough to keep us sober... We have gone through stages of dark despair when we were sure that something was wrong with us mentally... Today we are willing to accept the idea that, as far as we are concerned, alcoholism is an illness; a progressive illness that can never be "cured" but which, like some other illnesses, can be arrested. We agree that there is nothing shameful about having an illness, provided we face the problem honestly and try to do something about it. We are perfectly willing to admit that we are allergic to alcohol and that it is simply common sense to stay away from the source of the allergy.*

We understand now, that once a person has crossed the invisible line from heavy drinking to compulsive alcoholic drinking, they will always remain alcoholic. So far as we know, there can never be any turning back to "normal" social drinking. "Once an alcoholic - always an alcoholic" is a simple fact we have to live with.

We have also learned that there are few alternatives for the alcoholic. If they continue to drink, their problem will become progressively worse. They seem assuredly on the path to the gutter, to hospitals, to jails or other institutions, or to an early grave. The only alternative is to stop drinking completely and to abstain from even the smallest quantity of alcohol in any form. If they are willing to follow this course, and to take advantage of the help available to them, a whole new life can open up for the alcoholic."[134]

This language is confusing. Alcoholics Anonymous is asking the individual who needs help to accept that they have something wrong with them. The poor drinker has a "physical compulsion, coupled with a mental obsession," or has realised that "something was wrong with us mentally." Even more worrying is the potential that the drinker might have an illness. They may have to be "willing to admit that we are allergic to alcohol." For the drinker looking for insight this language misses the obvious. The problem doesn't lie with the individual, the problem is the substance, the alcohol. It is addictive and harmful. There is nothing wrong with the individual drinker - no illness, no allergy, no compulsion. The text includes this common sense advice though: "The only alternative is to stop drinking completely and to abstain from even the smallest quantity of alcohol in any form." which is sensible advice for all drinkers.

The doctrine of Alcoholics Anonymous also includes a dangerous and false

---

[134] About Alcoholism, Alcoholics Anonymous, https://www.alcoholics-anonymous.org.uk/ About-AA/Newcomers/About-Alcoholism [17.3.21]

stereotype in the definition of the alcoholic. In the text above is this frightening scenario: "once a person has crossed the invisible line from heavy drinking to compulsive alcoholic drinking, they will always remain alcoholic." There is a degree of truth in the definition. Individuals that drink heavily every day will find that alcohol is much more addictive than it was when they drank less. And this late stage pattern of drinking is the only way that they will be able to drink - heavy drinkers find it extremely difficult to moderate their intake.

Drinkers at this stage of the drinking journey will find that they are anxious all day, and consume large amounts of alcohol to try to alleviate the anxiety. But the cause of the condition is the amount of alcohol they drink, not an ailment. An alcoholic as defined by Alcoholics Anonymous is not diseased, doesn't have a condition, and hasn't caused a change to their brain function. Drinking heavily causes high levels of anxiety which leads to more drinking. Cutting down doesn't work, and Alcoholics Anonymous is right to say that the only option is to stop drinking.

It may be helpful to a heavy drinker to be labelled an alcoholic, and it is true that drinking heavily, or binge drinking, is compulsive. The stereotype of the alcoholic, and the way that AA defines it, though is dangerous to all other drinkers because of the message that it conveys. By labelling the individuals that need help as alcoholics, people who have "crossed the invisible line from heavy drinking to compulsive alcoholic drinking," they provide comfort to drinkers that feel they are not in this category. Drinkers that consider that their use of alcohol isn't compulsive, or that feel that they are in control of their drinking, as all drinkers do, have their drinking levels validated by the idea of the alcoholic. Drinkers can continue to drink, safe in the knowledge that they haven't "crossed the invisible line."

Dr Suzi Gage writing in *Say Why to Drugs* says,

> "...the term 'alcoholic' to describe people with alcohol dependence is

*falling out of favour... While some in the past have said that defining
alcohol problems as the disease 'alcoholism' can shift stigma away
from an individual, others fear that such labels are equally stigmatising,
implying 'rock bottom' and a lifelong diagnosis... As well as this the
term might create an 'othering' of problematic alcohol abuse, giving
some people like a get out clause – 'Oh well, my drinking isn't as bad
as that, I'm not an alcoholic so I don't need to do anything about my
drinking.'"*[135]

The other dangerous aspect of the label of alcoholic is to the people who have
concluded that they have become one and are now a lost cause, or beyond
help. Self identifying as a drinker that has crossed the invisible line may feel
that they are beyond help, and beyond making the effort to stop.

Here's TV host Chris Tarrant talking about his drinking in an interview with
the Guardian newspaper: "I don't drink whisky at all now. Nobody told me
not to," he says proudly. How much did he used to drink? "A lot. I liked it.
Neat." Could he get through a bottle in a day? "Not in an evening, no!" He
looks appalled. A half bottle? Now he looks insulted. "I'd get through a half
watching telly, oh God, yes. I was never crawling on the floor or drinking out
of dustbins. I was never an alcoholic... He admits there were times he feared
he was an alcoholic. So he checked himself out at the doctor's. "At the end
of the tests, they said you are not an alcoholic, but you're a heavy drinker.
Carry on like this and you may become one."[136] This is a perfect example of
the myth of the alcoholic and again shows how dangerous this thinking is.
Chris and Chris' doctor both seem to believe in the idea of the invisible line
that can be crossed from heavy drinker to alcoholic. Luckily both of them are

---

[135] Suzi Gage, *Say Why to Drugs*, Hodder & Stoughton, Jan 2020.

[136] Simon Hattenstone, *Chris Tarrant: 'We were less respectful of women, full stop'*, The Guardian,
https://www.theguardian.com/tv-and-radio/2018/oct/28/chris-tarrant-we-were-less-
respectful-of-women-full-stop [17.3.21]

sensible enough to realise that drinking half a bottle of whiskey is extremely bad for you. "You're not an alcoholic, you're just a heavy drinker."

Small amounts of alcohol are detrimental to our natural perfect selves. The more we consume, the more harm we do, and the more we drink over time, the more addictive the substance becomes. There isn't a line we cross where we suddenly become an alcoholic. The way that each drinker consumes alcohol is the result of the amount of alcohol they have consumed over time. Alcoholics Anonymous is right to say that the individuals that go to them for help cannot cut down. Drinkers in the later stages of their drinking find it increasingly difficult to cut down. The only option is to stop, but this advice shouldn't be restricted to its members. Every drinker should stop because all alcohol is harmful. The belief that drinking is fine and harmless, or that heavy drinking is fine, provided drinkers don't cross an invisible line, is dangerous.

The idea of the alcoholic is a big part of the myths that drinkers buy into. It colours the way drinkers think about drinking, believing they are in control, but that the poor unfortunate alcoholics have lost control. The myth is reinforced by the language and thinking of Alcoholics Anonymous, and it seems to be reinforced by the highly visible sight of the down and outs in the city centre. They drink every night, and they represent the definition of what an alcoholic is. They have clearly lost control, and their alcohol intake is visible for all to see. But the down and outs are a minority of the drinkers that make up the numbers of people in hospital wards and in the mortuaries.

The majority of the drinkers that suffer harm due to their intake are the wealthy grown ups that make up the professional classes. In a Guardian article entitled *Wealthy professionals most likely to drink regularly, figures show*, reporting studies from NHS Digital and the ONS, the article states:

> *"Data from previous years in the Health Survey for England showed the most harmful drinking was among middle-aged people, who were more likely to drink every day. "Middle-class drinkers are unlikely to*

pay attention to government health warnings as they may be less likely to get excessively drunk, and can withstand increases in prices," said Steve Clarke, an alcohol addiction therapy services manager with the Priory Group." The over-45s particularly are drinking more regularly but not thinking they're in danger. But they are drinking four, five, six days a week and it all adds up. In 2016-17 [in England] there were 337,000 estimated hospital admissions attributable to alcohol – that's a jump of 17%, nearly a fifth, on 2006-07," he said."[137]

Alcohol Policy UK states, "New research published in the British Medical Journal suggests being 'middle class' is linked to higher risk drinking amongst over 50s... The study found factors such as higher educational attainment, being socially active and good ratings of health were associated with higher risk drinking... Higher risk drinking, referred to as 'harmful drinking' in NICE guidelines, was defined by the study as drinking over 50 units per week in men and over 35 units per week in women."[138] Well educated, socially active, otherwise healthy drinkers, in their 50s and upwards are not what we typically think of as alcoholics. When we think of alcoholics we tend to think of the highly visible problem drinkers on the streets, drinking cheap super strength lager.

In a similar article *Regular binge drinking can cause long-term brain damage,* also in the Guardian the focus is on binge drinking, stating, "Just a few sessions of heavy drinking can damage someone's ability to pay attention, remember things and make good judgments, research shows... Binge drinkers aged between 18 and 24 are a key target of the government's alcohol strategy...

---

[137] Sarah Boseley, *Wealthy professionals most likely to drink regularly, figures show,* The Guardian, https://www.theguardian.com/society/2018/may/01/wealthy-professionals-most-likely-to-drink-alcohol-regularly-figures-show [17.3.21]

[138] *Middle class' middle age drinkers most at risk,* Alcohol Policy UK, https://www.alcoholpolicy.net/2015/07/middle-class-middle-age-drinkers-at-higher-risk.html, [17.3.21]

Professor Ian Gilmore, president of the Royal College of Physicians, said: "We know large numbers of people in this country binge drink. This should be a wake-up call to the millions of people whose lifestyle means they get drunk regularly."[139] Young binge drinkers are another group that we wouldn't think of as typical alcoholics but they are clearly causing themselves harm via their intake.

This Guardian article, Binge-drink Britain: how one weekend bender can ruin your life, highlights the damage that drinkers can cause to their pancreas, describing a number of drinkers, who "developed pancreatitis, a disease brought on by excessive alcohol consumption that can turn one night in the pub, or a day at the beach, into a life-altering illness – it can often be fatal."[140] Again, this is damage brought on by binge drinking and can affect anyone at any age. Every drinker that has caused themselves damage in a heavy drinking session knew for certain that they hadn't crossed an invisible line to become an alcoholic, and believed naively that their intake would not cause them serious harm.

The messaging and the myth that is the result of Alcoholics Anonymous' definition contributes to drinking harm, in the groups of drinkers that feel their drinking is normal and under control, and this means all drinkers. The individuals that die or harm themselves most are the same people that would never associate themselves with Alcoholics Anonymous' definitions. If at any time in their drinking journey, these individuals spent time on the Alcoholics Anonymous website to try to get a sense of the risks they were taking, they would find little clarity. Regular drinkers from the professional classes don't feel they have crossed an invisible line and developed a compulsion.

---

[139] Denis Campbell, *Regular binge drinking can cause long-term brain damage - study*, The Guardian, https://www.theguardian.com/society/2008/dec/29/binge-drinking-brain-damage-study [17.3.21]

[140] Sirin Kale, *Binge-drink Britain: how one weekend bender can ruin your life*, The Guardian, https://www.theguardian.com/lifeandstyle/2018/may/30/one-weekend-bender-can-ruin-your-life-pancreatitis [17.3.21]

27

Alcoholism and alcohol use disorder

I had an afternoon social in a pub with a couple of friends recently. I was drinking lime and soda. The two friends were drinking pints of cider. At some point the conversation came round to my beliefs about alcohol and I mentioned alcoholism and was about to start telling the friends that I didn't believe in it but before I had a chance my friend's wife said "that's what my sister died of. Alcoholism." There was a pause, and she carried on drinking cider.

Alcoholism features in the literature of Alcoholics Anonymous and has become part of the way we talk about problem drinking but it isn't a disease or a physical or mental condition. Doctors can't do a blood test to find an infection or a virus. There isn't a change to the brain that can be measured to tell if you have contracted it. Because alcohol is addictive, some people drink enough alcohol to harm themselves, and some of them die because of the amount of alcohol they have consumed. This isn't alcoholism, it is alcohol. My friend's sister (she's in her mid-30s) didn't die of alcoholism, she died because she drank too much alcohol. Alcohol killed her, not a disease called alcoholism.

Obviously for my friend, it was inconvenient to say that alcohol killed her sister, especially when she was halfway through a pint of cider. Every drinker finds it difficult to acknowledge that the alcohol they drink day to day, that they believe fuels their socialising and provides relaxation, is the same alcohol that harms and kills other drinkers. Alcohol kills people, not alcoholism. Alcohol kills 5% of the worlds' population every year. That is 1 in 20 people. That one person out of every 20 didn't catch a mysterious illness called alcoholism, they just drank too much of the poisonous, addictive drug that my friends were enjoying in the pub. The World Health Organization says, "Alcohol consumption is a causal factor in more than 200 disease and injury conditions. Drinking alcohol is associated with a risk of developing health problems such as mental and behavioural disorders, including alcohol dependence, major noncommunicable diseases such as liver cirrhosis, some cancers and cardiovascular diseases."[141] Not alcoholism, alcohol.

Here is a muddled definition: "Alcoholism is the most severe form of alcohol abuse and involves the inability to manage drinking habits. It is also commonly referred to as alcohol use disorder. Alcohol use disorder is organized into three categories: mild, moderate and severe. Each category has various symptoms and can cause harmful side effects. If left untreated, any type of alcohol abuse can spiral out of control."[142] This is an interesting text because not only is the mystery alcoholism defined as an inability to manage drinking habits, the Alcohol Rehab Guide splits into three categories, and suggests treatment. The treatment is to stop drinking. The problem is alcohol. Problem use of an addictive drug is not a habit, it is an addiction.

The number of news stories, personal posts online and websites that repeat the myth that somebody died of alcoholism is huge. "My husband died of alcoholism and his family are blaming me for abandoning him."[143] "his

---

[141] *Alcohol,* World Health Organization, https://www.who.int/news-room/fact-sheets/detail/alcohol [17.3.21]

[142] Carol Galbicsek, *What is Alcoholism?,* Alcohol Rehab Guide, https://www.alcoholrehabguide.org/alcohol/ [17.3.21]

[143] Deidre Sanders, *Bereaved by Booze My husband died of alcoholism and now his family blame me for his death,* The Sun, https://www.thesun.co.uk/dear-deidre/10128813/late-husband-alcoholism-death/ [17.3.21]

mother, who died of alcoholism when he was 16."[144] "told how she will spend another Christmas without her dad Gerry, who died of alcoholism."[145] Three examples among thousands and thousands. Drinkers don't like to see these deaths as being attributed to alcohol and prefer to believe in the imaginary condition, falsely distinguishing between drinkers who believe they are in control, and drinkers that have lost control.

We don't apply the same type of language to users of other addictive substances. Should we describe the smokers that end up causing themselves to contract COPD or lung cancer as suffering from nicotinism? Or tobaccoism? These smokers have consumed an addictive toxic drug. The tobacco they smoked has harmed them in the same way that the alcohol harms drinkers. We don't label heroin addicts that overdose as having a condition or an illness called opiateism or heroinism. They didn't die of opiateism, heroin killed them. We accept that use of opiates tends to increase over time and we know how addictive this class of drugs can be. Powder cocaine and crack cocaine can cause all sorts of health problems and can lead to death. The users that die taking the drug don't die of cocaineism. They die because cocaine is poisonous and if a user takes enough it has the potential to kill.

It sounds blunt to say "my mum died from drinking", or "alcohol killed my best friend," but this is the truth. An addictive drug, alcohol, caused the user to drink and drink until they suffered harm or died. This is what alcohol does to people that don't exercise restraint.

Alcohol use disorder is a similar term that continues the myth of us and them, the drinkers that feel they are in control, as opposed to the drinkers that have lost control. The term is used by experts that drink to describe problem

---

[144] *Booker Prize 2020: Douglas Stuart's novel Shuggie Bain wins*, BBC News, https://www.bbc.co.uk/news/entertainment-arts-54976523 [17.3.21]

[145] Mark McGivern, *Heartbreaking candlelit vigil held in Glasgow to remember 1187 drug deaths before election hustings*, Daily Record, https://www.dailyrecord.co.uk/news/scottish-news/heartbreaking-candlelit-vigil-held-glasgow-21041968 [17.3.21]

drinkers. Again, we don't describe a smoking use disorder or an opiate use disorder. All use of an addictive harmful drug is a disorder. Some smoking is a disorder. If you smoke 10 a day you are not in control of your smoking, and you wouldn't describe a 20 a day smoker as having a smoking disorder.

Agencies that inform the public about alcohol seem undecided if alcohol use disorder is a psychiatric condition. The study, *Psychiatric comorbidities in alcohol use disorder*, says, "Alcohol use disorder is a major contributor to the morbidity and mortality burden worldwide. It often coexists with other psychiatric disorders; however, the nature of this comorbidity is still a matter of debate."[146] This uncertainty is understandable. Medical professionals treat patients that drink and have mental health conditions, and some of those drinkers drink heavily. Are they mentally ill because the alcohol has damaged their healthy mind, or was there an underlying health condition that led them to drink more? It is well known that alcohol causes a range of mental health conditions and that heavy drinkers have high anxiety levels, sometimes chaotic lives and poor sleep. It shouldn't be a surprise that drinking leads to cognitive damage. If the professionals that treat individuals who suffer the effects of heavy drinking though are also drinkers they may be reluctant to accept that the substance they consume, and that seems relatively harmless to them, has inflicted psychological damage.

Both the terms "alcohol use disorder", and "alcoholism" are prevalent in the debate and advice around alcohol, and cloud our understanding of alcohol. Both terms offer a false explanation for the harm that alcohol can inflict. The terms shift the blame away from alcohol, and allow drinkers that consider their intake to be normal, to continue to drink, believing that they are not in danger. Experts will point to the fact that both terms are used to describe what they would call compulsive drinking but this, like the idea of the alcoholic,

---

[146] Alvaro Castillo-Carniglia et al. *Psychiatric comorbidities in alcohol use disorder,* The Lancet, https://www.thelancet.com/journals/lanpsy/article/PIIS2215-0366(19)30222-6/ [17.3.21]

reinforces the idea of a line that is crossed, when normal drinking becomes compulsive. Each drinker at the later stages of their drinking journey has experienced the same stages between their first drink and their current intake, moving from first drinking experience to social drinking, more regular drinking, daily drinking, heavy daily drinking, etc. Alcohol causes users to increase their drinking because it becomes more addictive. There isn't a line when drinkers suddenly find that their alcohol use has become compulsive, it has always been a compulsion, albeit one that has got more controlling the more that they consume.

Here's an interesting point from the Guardian, "The term alcoholism has long been retired from official alcohol clinical and policy guidance, abandoned as a reductionist and stigmatising label for problem drinking. Instead, alcohol use disorders, some including varying degrees of dependency, reflect the wider continuum nature of alcohol problems."[147] Aren't they almost the same thing though? Each one is an invented condition to describe someone who is a heavy drinker. No heavy drinker drinks what they do of their own free will. Nobody ever decided out of the blue that as of this moment, they would start drinking two bottles of wine every night. Heavy drinking is the result of moderate drinking, and a failure to exercise restraint. Increased consumption creeps up on drinkers and can typically take years or decades after the first drinking experience. The extra free time and financial freedom brought on by retirement, or by the kids leaving the family home means that it is more of a problem as people get older. The quote is correct though describing the "continuum nature of alcohol problems."

---

[147] James Morris, *The media has a problem with alcoholism – and it's stopping people getting help*, The Guardian, https://www.theguardian.com/science/sifting-the-evidence/2017/nov/22/the-media-has-a-problem-with-alcoholism [17.3.21]

28

The blame

The alcohol industry and Alcoholics Anonymous share a common feature, which is surprising given they have opposing aims. The corporations that sell alcohol exist to deliver profit to their shareholders, an easy job when the product they sell is addictive. Alcoholics Anonymous exists to support problem drinkers that have been harmed by alcohol, or allowed alcohol to exert control over them. These two organisations should have a philosophy that is in direct conflict but they each share a belief that the drinker is to blame for alcohol addiction. Alcoholics Anonymous labels drinkers that come to them for help as alcoholics, and asks them to accept they have a disease called alcoholism. The problem lies with the drinker, and the drinker needs to accept that they are flawed in some way. They have crossed an invisible line and there is no going back. Alcoholics Anonymous does not tell its members that the substance in the bottle is a poisonous addictive drug that has the power to exert control over everybody that consumes it. The blame for consumption sits squarely on the shoulders of the drinker.

The alcohol industry likes to explain problem drinking away by blaming the drinkers that suffer harm as being problem users. EUCAM describes this as in its report *Seven Key Messages of the Alcohol Industry*, as "The Damage Done by Alcohol is Caused by a Small Group of Deviants Who Cannot Handle Alcohol," saying, "The image communicated by the industry: It is only a small group of individuals who abuse alcohol that cause problems such as crime, the spread of diseases, staff absenteeism, violence, sexual abuse and poverty. They are abusers of alcohol who must be dealt with individually. It is symbolic politics to think we can eliminate these problems by collective measures. Moreover, such measures would penalize the majority of individuals who are responsible consumers of alcohol."[148] In short, don't blame alcohol, blame the drinkers.

EUCAM goes on to say, "[The alcohol industry believes] it is not the alcohol that is the problem, but the irresponsible behaviour of this group of drinkers that is highlighted as the cause of the above mentioned problems. The fact that the majority of individuals who consume high levels of alcohol are in fact ordinary, everyday citizens who are not social deviants is not the message the alcohol industry presents. Indeed, the message of the industry is that ordinary citizens drink responsibly and that 'bad' citizens drink irresponsibly and are the cause of any and all problems associated with high alcohol consumption. In reality the alcohol industry earns millions of euros on heavy drinkers. The industry claims that their marketing efforts only result in the 'responsible consumption of alcohol', but If that were indeed the case, the profits of the alcohol industry would plummet enormously."[149] Not only does the industry label the drinkers as bad apples, it also earns much of its income from these individuals. The more the drinker drinks, the more addictive the alcohol becomes, and the more harm the drinkers cause to themselves and the people around them. At the same time they spend more and more on booze.

Alcoholics Anonymous and the alcohol industry both blame drinkers for very different reasons. The industry doesn't want us to see its overpriced product as a poisonous addictive drug, because then we wouldn't buy it. AA presents the problem of alcohol addiction in the simplest possible way for its community of ex-drinkers, and for lack of a better explanation uses the label of alcoholic, and the invented disease of alcoholism to make it clear

---

[148] *Seven Key Messages of the Alcohol Industry,* EUCAM

[149] *Seven Key Messages of the Alcohol Industry,* EUCAM

to its members that they need to abstain. These ideas have permeated the way we collectively think about alcohol and are accepted and repeated by drinkers. Alcoholics Anonymous is in a prime position to be an opponent of the alcohol industry. The charity could use its power and influence to highlight the danger of the drug that the corporations sell, but instead the focus is on the individual that has lost control. This suits the alcohol industry perfectly and even supports their argument that a few deviants or bad apples are responsible for the harm. Instead of countering the alcohol industry Alcoholics Anonymous supports its views.

29

Medical language

We describe drinkers that have stopped drinking in medical terms that reinforce the idea that alcoholics, or those that we believe have suffered from alcoholism, have suffered from a medical condition or a disease. The phraseology has been borrowed from the world of medicine and relates to the treatment of diseases. We describe drinkers that have stopped drinking as "alcoholics in recovery". "In recovery" originated to describe patients that have recently been treated or operated on, and we talk about cancer patients being in recovery post-treatment. In fact an "alcoholic in recovery" is someone who used to drink, and has stopped drinking because the alcohol they consumed negatively affected them.

A "cure" for alcoholism is a common term that is often repeated and it is included in a number of book titles that focus on ways to control alcohol intake. When we stop drinking we haven't cured anything. There has been no disease, and therefore no cure. The decision to stop drinking alcohol is just that, and is normally based on the realisation that alcohol is a detrimental, harmful substance. When an ex-drinker makes a mistake and drinks alcohol again, we describe this as a "relapse", another term borrowed from the world of medicine. A relapse is a deterioration after a period of improvement and typically refers to a patient suffering a disease or medical condition. Less common is the term "in remission," used here: "The aim of this study was to examine longitudinal changes in recovery status among individuals in remission from... alcohol dependence,"[150] which again describes drinkers that have stopped drinking, and originated from the field of cancer treatment.

Each of these medical terms originated in the biased guidance produced by experts. This guidance has informed the way that we collectively think about drinking alcohol. Medical terms to describe problem drinking shift the blame for the harm that is caused by drinking away from alcohol, and onto the individual drinkers. Because the experts drink alcohol, they are reluctant to blame their own favourite tipple, and instead have invented terms such as alcoholic to describe heavy drinkers, or drinkers that harm themselves. They make up diseases and conditions called alcoholism, alcohol use disorder, and alcohol dependence syndrome to imply that the made-up disease has caused harm rather than the alcohol. They have borrowed the language of medical practice to continue the deceit. No other addictive drug gets the same treatment. The public, the media and drinkers repeat these terms without stopping to think if they are real, and valid, and the repetition further embeds them.

Ex-drinkers don't need to label themselves or think of themselves as having been afflicted by a disease. Alcohol is the problem, and when drinkers realise this, and stop drinking they just become a non-drinker. Rather than using medical language I describe my own experience of alcohol as: I used to drink, it was bad for me, I stopped. I definitely drank too much. This is simple language and true. I didn't drink a benign substance only to find that I was unlucky enough to develop a disease called alcoholism, which I then had to cure, and thankfully I am now in recovery. This nonsense obscures the truth about alcohol, that it is addictive and harmful. Alcohol is the problem.

---

[150] Deborah Dawson et al. *Rates and Correlates of Relapse Among Individuals in Remission From DSM-IV Alcohol Dependence: A 3-Year Follow-Up*, January 2008 Alcoholism Clinical and Experimental Research, ResearchGate, https://www.researchgate.net/publication/5812360 [17.3.21]

30

Conclusion

In 1964 the Advisory Committee to the Surgeon General in the US issued a report, *Smoking and Health*, which stated clearly that tobacco smoke causes lung cancer. At the time smoking was widespread in the US and "crossed socioeconomic, gender, race, and ethnicity boundaries. Cigarette smoking was widely accepted, highly prevalent, and not discouraged in homes, and it took place in public spaces of all kinds, including hospitals, restaurants, airplanes, and medical conferences."[151] The Surgeon General's report marked a turning point in American tobacco consumption and started to make it clear in the mind of the public that smoking cigarettes causes cancer. Since the report was published smoking rates have steadily declined in the US from 40% of the population to around 20%.[152]

In 1965 the tobacco companies voluntarily accepted a warning label which would be added to cigarette packets: "Caution: Cigarette Smoking May Be Hazardous to Your Health." The softening of this message says a lot about the influence of the tobacco companies of the time. The Surgeon General's report

---

[151] *The Health Consequences of Smoking—50 Years of Progress: A Report of the Surgeon General*, National Center for Chronic Disease Prevention and Health Promotion (US) Office on Smoking and Health, https://www.ncbi.nlm.nih.gov/books/NBK294310/ [17.3.21]

[152] *The Health Consequences of Smoking—50 Years of Progress: A Report of the Surgeon General*,

said quite clearly that tobacco smoke causes lung cancer. Cigarette smoking is definitely hazardous to health, but the tobacco companies helpfully explained to smokers that it "may be" hazardous. This is one example of the efforts of the tobacco sellers to counter what is obvious to us all now, that tobacco is dangerous and addictive. The US Government's efforts at the time to improve public health included issuing public information that aimed to help smokers reduce the harm of smoking including advising them to choose cigarettes with less tar, smoking less of the cigarette, or smoking fewer cigarettes. This type of messaging had limited impact but suited the tobacco industry in that it didn't tell smokers to stop. It took years for the messages about lung cancer to become part of the public understanding: "It was not until the 1970s that a majority of Americans said smoking was a cause of lung cancer. But the proportion with this view climbed steadily from about 70% during the 1970s to about 80% in the 1980s. By the 1990s, Gallup polls consistently showed 95% of Americans claiming to believe cigarette smoking to be harmful to health and 90% believing it to be a cause of lung cancer."[153]

The tobacco industry, and attitudes to smoking in the mid-60s has parallels with the alcohol industry now, and our current consumption of alcohol. Compared to the way that the Government controls and restricts the tobacco industry it seems that its regulation of the alcohol industry is about 50 years behind. Tobacco and alcohol are both carcinogenic addictive drugs that have made huge profits for a small group of powerful corporations. Tobacco producers of the time and alcohol suppliers now are equally reluctant to accept controls, and both groups lobby Governments to prevent outright bans on their product. Their marketing efforts involved huge spending to present an addictive toxic drug as a glamorous and sophisticated product. Hollywood stars that smoked were once seen as cool and interesting, in the same way a number of screen icons now are presented as glamorous and sophisticated consumers of alcohol. In the 60s, "cigarette smoking was widely accepted, highly prevalent, and not discouraged in homes, and it took place in public

---

[153] *The Health Consequences of Smoking—50 Years of Progress: A Report of the Surgeon General,*

spaces of all kinds, including hospitals, restaurants, airplanes, and medical conferences." as drinking is now.

The users of each drug have a set of mistaken beliefs that allow them to continue consuming the drug, even though each use of the drug is unpleasant. Smokers and drinkers both argue that their drug of choice is relaxing, and relieves stress. We are all well aware that tobacco smoke causes cancer, and we should also be aware that drinking alcohol does the same. The numbers of people that suffer harm from smoking is huge. "Tobacco smoking is one of the world's largest health problems... It has been a major health problem for many decades. For the entire 20th century it is estimated that around 100 million people died prematurely because of smoking, most of them in rich countries."[154] The WHO suggests that 3 million die every year from drinking alcohol[155], the equivalent of 300 million over the course of a century. Tobacco use and alcohol use both cross ethnic, gender and socio-economic boundaries. Smokers make up a cross-section of the public, as do drinkers.

In the UK now, cigarette use is actively discouraged with very tight controls, including packets of cigarettes hidden in shops, photos of cancer and medical injuries on packets, bans on advertising and advice from our experts to stop smoking. Alcohol is treated very differently with far less control imposed on advertising, no warning labels and advice from experts encouraging us to drink in moderation. The messaging and guidance that the experts provide to us mirrors the advice given out during the 60s in the US to reduce tobacco harm, with a blanket refusal to condemn alcohol. Books, websites, health practitioners and the press cannot seem to tell us what is obvious, that alcohol is harmful and that we should not consume it. Instead we are told again and again to cut down. Just like the advice to smokers to smoke less, this advice is

---

[154] Hannah Ritchie and Max Roser, *Smoking*, Our World in Data, https://ourworldindata.org/smoking [17.3.21]

[155] *Alcohol*, World Health Organization, https://www.who.int/news-room/fact-sheets/detail/alcohol [17.3.21]

dangerous.

In 1964 around 40% of Americans were smokers. According to the Office of National Statistics, "In 2017, among adults aged 16 years and over, 57.0% of respondents drank alcohol in the week before being interviewed for the Opinions and Lifestyle Survey. This equates to 29.2 million people in the population of Great Britain." Around 14% of adults in the UK smoke cigarettes.[156] Comparing US tobacco use of the 60s to the way that tobacco is consumed today, it is clear that the effort by Government to bring down the numbers of smokers has worked. In the UK, restrictions on tobacco advertising, removal of in-store displays of cigarettes, removal of branding from packages, and messaging focused on stopping smoking has resulted in reduced tobacco use. The wide restrictions combined with clear public messaging have had an impact. Smoking now is out of favour among the public, who largely welcomed the ban on smoking in public places in 2007.

A key aspect of the guidance and messaging around smoking is the unambiguous message that tobacco is harmful, and that we should not smoke. We don't see vague and conflicting guidance advising smokers to try to have smoke-free days, or to reduce their intake to 14 cigarettes a week. Nobody would tell us now that tobacco is pleasurable or relaxing and that we should smoke in moderation. The guidance issued by the NHS does not say that moderation of tobacco is fine, but that harmful use of tobacco is bad. The guidance does not split smokers into two groups, the "normal" smokers who think they are in control, and the ones who have lost control. It's language is clear: "Every year around 78,000 people in the UK die from smoking, with many more living with debilitating smoking-related illnesses... Smoking increases your risk of developing more than 50 serious health conditions... Some may be fatal, and

---

[156] *Adult smoking habits in the UK: 2018*, Office for National Statistics, https://www.ons.gov.uk/ peoplepopulationandcommunity/healthandsocialcare/healthandlifeexpectancies/ bulletins/adultsmokinghabitsingreatbritain/2018 [17.3.21]

others can cause irreversible long-term damage to your health."[157]

Over the last few decades our attitudes to smoking have changed, and this has been brought about by Government efforts to restrict the power of the tobacco companies, in order to benefit the health of the nation. This is not mirrored in Government efforts to restrict the power of the alcohol companies. In future we may see Government messaging that tells us clearly that alcohol is addictive and harmful, that it is toxic to humans and causes cancer. We may be told not to drink it. We may see advertising and sponsorship restricted, branding curtailed, and the displays in supermarkets hidden away as they are for cigarettes. These restrictions, and clearer guidance will lead to improved public health, less harm and less cost to the NHS.

There is evidence though that the younger generations tend to drink less. The BBC reported, "Researchers looked at official health data from the last decade and found almost a third of 16 to 24-year-olds in 2015 said they didn't drink, compared with around one in five in 2005...Non-drinking was found across a broad range of groups, suggesting it was becoming "more mainstream."[158] Sales of low alcohol and alcohol-free beers are increasing year on year. Miles Beale, chief executive of the Wine and Spirit Trade Association said, "The low-alcohol wine category has increased 10 times since 2009 to around 3% of the market – that's more than 37 million bottles, worth over £70m. Producers are responding to consumer demand for products that fit changing lifestyle habits – we know that overall alcohol consumption is decreasing, particularly among young people – with innovative new products that are lower in alcohol."[159]

---

[157] *What are the health risks of smoking?*, NHS, https://www.nhs.uk/common-health-questions/lifestyle/what-are-the-health-risks-of-smoking/ [17.3.21]

[158] *Under-25s turning their backs on alcohol, study suggests*, BBC News, https://www.bbc.co.uk/news/uk-45807152 [17.3.21]

[159] Rebecca Smithers, *Millennials make it a slow booze summer in the UK*, The Guardian, https://www.theguardian.com/society/2018/jun/23/slow-booze-summer-millennials-low-alcohol-drinks [17.3.21]

For now we must accept that there is an unwillingness by the Government to control the sale of alcohol in any meaningful way, and that the alcohol industry wields serious power, which will allow it to continue making money from massive numbers of drinkers. Each individual though has the freedom to abstain from alcohol, and to reject the pressure to drink. Nobody has to consume alcohol. We know deep down that it goes against nature, that it is bad for us, that it can kill us, and we all have experience of the harm that it can cause in friends and loved ones that have suffered harm. Although alcohol is highly addictive we can each be free of it by changing our beliefs about the substance and recognising that we are mistaken about the benefits of drinking it.

Any drinker that can see past the peer pressure, the marketing that focuses on glamour and sophistication, and that decides to see alcohol for what it really is will find it easy to be free of it. A drinker that has regularly consumed alcohol will feel anxious and edgy when they stop, but this is the effect of the stress hormone cortisol in their system, and over the course of a few days this will dissipate, leaving the drinker relaxed and content as every non-drinker is, with more time, more money, increased energy and improved happiness.

Every drinker can remember the time when he or she became a drinker. In our early drinking experiences we had to learn to poison ourselves, egged on by our fellow drinkers. There is nothing natural about drinking something that smells bad, that tastes nasty and that causes our natural reflexes to vomit out the substance to keep us safe. When we slurred our words, lost control of our coordination or injured ourselves, were we each making ourselves into sophisticated, suave, classy people, or were we just conditioning our poor natural amazing bodies to tolerate a toxic substance? Did we have to overcome our natural controls and safety mechanism in order to allow alcohol to control us? Was it really in our best interests to "acquire the taste", and to allow other drinkers to tell us what is good for us? Should we have listened to the warning signs that nature gave us? Are we better as adults that regularly poison ourselves with overpriced rotten grape juice, or should we remember what we were like as kids, 100% natural social creatures without a drink in our hand.

When each of us thinks back over our drinking life, have we improved ourselves, made ourselves happier, impressed our peers, charmed members of the opposite sex or had amazing social experiences because of the alcohol, or in spite of it. Would we have been happier without alcohol, would our natural charm and wit have impressed our friends without the influence of booze? Would we have been more charming, better flirts, great conversationalists and perfect social creatures without needing to anesthetise ourselves? Would we have been more in control, funnier, and better at keeping our emotions in check? Would we have maintained relationships and friendships, been better at work, achieved our goals, and improved ourselves further if we hadn't drunk alcohol?

Each drinker should also be aware of their current position on the drinking journey, and recognise that they didn't arrive at that point through free choice. Each drinker did not start out drinking at the same level they consume now. Nobody planned to drink as much as they do now. Every drinker progresses along the line, drinking more and more. Because this progress happens over an extended time it's not until each drinker stops to consider their drinking with detachment that they recognise that the level they drink at now is not a free choice. This aspect of giving up control to an addictive drug, succumbing to the addictive properties of alcohol makes every drinker less happy. My friend who gave up drinking told me she felt smug every night she was out. She behaved better, she slept better, she left the pub or restaurant at a good time, and she woke up feeling fresh and energetic every morning. Should we feel smug when we finally understand that alcohol is not a positive aspect of our lives and make the decision to stop drinking it? Damn right we should. All non-drinkers are more in control of their lives than drinkers, they are more satisfied and enjoy more freedom. There is a lot to be smug about.

Drinkers are not in control and they are not free. The beliefs that alcohol is part of social interaction, that it is a necessary part of the restaurant experience, and that it is essential for celebrating with friends, are myths. These ideas are constantly reinforced by the massive army of drinkers that don't want individuals to break rank. Drinkers don't drink because it makes them happy, or because it makes them interesting, or because it benefits them in any way. They drink because alcohol is addictive. When a drinker rejects these beliefs and makes the decision to be free of alcohol he or she will experience a new found freedom. A friend and client who drank two bottles of wine every night for most of her adult life told me after she had stopped drinking in her early 50s she felt free. One month after stopping she reported that her life had changed for the better and she was excited about feeling liberated. She was free of the need to drink every night, free of the controlling nature of alcohol that had previously caused her to drink glass after glass, trying to chase away an anxiety that she now knows was caused by the alcohol. Drinkers that stop by changing their beliefs about alcohol have no need to feel deprived of alcohol, and will not miss the substance.

Printed in Great Britain
by Amazon

56697835R00099